Evaluation of Nutrition Education in Africa

Communications 6

AFRIKA-STUDIECENTRUM · LEIDEN

JAN HOORWEG AND IAN McDOWELL

Evaluation of Nutrition Education in Africa

Community Research in Uganda, 1971–1972

MOUTON PUBLISHERS
THE HAGUE · PARIS · NEW YORK

The Afrika-Studiecentrum cannot in any way be held responsible for the views or opinions expressed in this publication.

Cover-design by Jurriaan Schrofer
ISBN: 90-279-7617-1

Printed in the Netherlands

Acknowledgements

The studies reported in this monograph were carried out in Uganda between early 1971 and the ominous summer of 1972. During this period we were lucky to be part of the staff of Makerere University, and it is sad that this stimulating intellectual community has since perished.

The studies were made possible by a grant, no. 651, from the Makerere Research Fund and also by the continuous support of Prof. Peter Rigby. Prof. J. Paget Stanfield helped us in many invaluable ways. Dr. Roger Whitehead, director of the Child Nutrition Unit of the Medical Research Council in Kampala, despite his healthy mistrust of social scientists, gave us material assistance, and we wish to thank our many friends among the former staff of that unit for their encouragement and support.

The studies would not have been possible without the lasting co-operation of the staff members at the Mwanamugimu and Luteete clinics. We admire their patience towards two curious and sometimes exasperating researchers and their assistants. We also appreciate the co-operation of the staff and students of the secondary schools and teacher training colleges at Namilyango, Namagunga, Ndejje, Nkozi, Busuubizi, and Namutamba. Without our assistants, Mrs. Janet Kabanda, Mrs. I. Kasirye, and Miss Francis Nabukenya, we would have been helpless. They were prepared to work irregular hours and to travel perilously over long distances, and they handled the interview situations with care and tact. We also thank John Orley for the data which he collected for us within the context of his own research.

The analysis of the data and the writing of this monograph took place after we had left Uganda and was made possible by our respective university departments, the Afrika-Studiecentrum at Leiden, and the Department of Community Health at the University of Nottingham. Rudo Niemeijer provided statistical advice and computer assistance, although he is not to be held responsible for any statistical shortcomings. Margaret Nganga Waiyaki typed the various drafts of this monograph with great patience and care.

Nairobi/
Nottingham

Jan Hoorweg
Ian McDowell

Contents

Acknowledgements	5
List of tables and figures	9
Introduction	13
1. Protein-energy malnutrition in Uganda	19
2. Mwanamugimu and Luteete clinics	35
3. Evaluative research	46
4. Three nutrition programmes. First studies: method	57
5. Three nutrition programmes. First studies: results	66
6. A closer look at food preferences	76
7. Teacher training colleges	88
8. Environment and recovery I	94
9. Environment and recovery II	104
10. Conclusions	117
Appendix A. Measuring recovery rate	127
Appendix B. Measuring knowledge and attitudes	132
Notes	147
References	153

List of Tables and Figures

Tables

1. Nutrient content of various foodstuffs 21
2. The content of the education at Mwanamugimu nutrition rehabilitation centre 38
3. Long-term progress at Luteete 45
4. Study 1. Characteristics of first and regular attenders at Mwanamugimu and Luteete 58
5. Study 1. Characteristics of experimental and control groups after omission of selected cases 59
6. Knowledge scales 61
7. Study 1. Mean scores (and standard deviations) for control groups 66
8. Study 1. Mwanamugimu inpatients: Differences between experimental and control groups 68
9. Study 1. Mwanamugimu outpatients: Differences between experimental and control groups 69
10. Study 1. Mwanamugimu outpatients: Differences between experimental and control groups by tribe 69
11. Study 1. Luteete outpatients: Differences between experimental and control groups 70
12. Study 1. Mean scores (and standard deviations) for experimental groups 71
13. Study 1. Mean scores (and standard deviations) for Mwanamugimu staff 72
14. Study 1. Average weight/weight for age (percentage) in different outpatient groups 73

15. Study 1. Spearman rank correlations of knowledge and attitude scales with nutritional 'outcome' (outpatients) 74
16. Study 2. Characteristics of inpatient and outpatient groups 77
17. Study 2. Meals included in paired-comparison schedule 78
18. Study 2. Average number of choices for individual meals 79
19. Study 2. Preference matrix: Differences between experimental and control groups 81
20. Study 2. Outpatients: Mean scores (and standard deviations) for protein index and staple index 82
21. Study 2. Preference matrix: Differences between experimental and control groups, four comparisons combined 83
22. Study 2. Inpatients: Mean scores (and standard deviations) for protein index and staple index 84
23. Study 2. Inpatients: Mean scores on protein index and staple index for Baganda and other tribes 84
24. Study 3. Composition of different groups of students at teacher training colleges 89
25. Study 3. Mean scores (and standard deviations) for students at teacher training colleges 90
26. Data recorded on the case files at Mwanamugimu N.R.C. 97
27. Study 4. Average recovery scores for urban cases compared with rural cases, by tribe and family 100
28. Study 5. Single and multiple correlations of different socio-economic variables with recovery 111
29. Mean recovery values for young children compared with older children by formulae 2 and 3 129
30. Knowledge questions 133
31. Average number of choices for each of six staple foods 135
32. Average number of choices for each of six sauces 136
33. Average number of choices for each of six meals 137
34. Kruskal multidimensional scaling, 23 wordpairs: 4 dimensions 140
35. Semantic differential: Varimax rotation of first two principal components 143
36. Spearman rank correlations between knowledge and attitude scales 145

Figures

1. Uganda: regions and districts 18
2. Pretest-posttest control group design 51
3. Posttest-only control group design 55
4. Study 4. Average recovery score for different groups 102
5. The influence of the social environment on outpatient recovery from malnutrition 105
6. Semantic differential: Ratings of groups of villagers and nurses 142
7. Semantic differential: Frequency distributions of four composite scores 144

Introduction

Protein-energy malnutrition of early childhood is widely prevalent in many parts of the developing world. Research over the past twenty years has resulted in improved treatment and a greater understanding of the aetiology of the condition and has also resulted in an increased concern with the less conspicuous forms of malnutrition. In tropical Africa, for example, the children suffering from these less severe, but chronic, forms are many times more numerous than those showing acute syndromes. The past twenty years have also witnessed a growing concern with the consequences of malnutrition. These include not only high treatment costs but also increased child mortality, impaired physical and mental development, and immeasurable misery and suffering. It is now well established that childhood malnutrition is not limited to times of famine, to barren areas, or to impoverished groups. There exist endemic causes of malnutrition which affect the majority of children in many countries. These causes lie in a combination of health conditions, diet, and child-rearing practices.

The growing understanding of the endemic nature of childhood malnutrition led to a reassessment of the most suitable form of care. Instead of just treating acute cases in hospital, interest in many developing countries has focused on combining care with prevention. A major example of this trend is the creation of nutrition rehabilitation centres (N.R.C.s) which fulfil two main functions. They provide care for young children suffering from mild or moderate degrees of malnutrition and they educate mothers on how best to apply their limited resources in feeding their children. In this way they combine curative with preventive activities, in an endeavour to overcome the readmission of old cases and to prevent new cases from occurring. Mothers attend the centres regularly with their children and receive teaching on the dietary requirements of young children, on recommended foods, and often on child rearing in general. However, the work of the N.R.C.s is not unique; prevention through education is provided also by other programmes that seek to contact children at risk *before* they show symptoms of malnutrition. Examples are the education provided by maternal and child health clinics, by social workers in the cities, and by community development programmes in the rural areas.

There have been repeated demands for the evaluation of these activities. The evaluation that has been reported has been concerned mostly with curative, rather than preventive, aspects, and often compares the N.R.C.s with hospital care. Usually such studies assess the progress of the children by using anthropometric measures (Beghin and Viteri, 1973). From such data it has been claimed that these centres 'make a solid contribution' to the problems of undernutrition (King, 1970, p. 307). Other authors are more equivocal because nearly everywhere a persistent minority of children fail to recover their weight deficit despite continued attendance (Bengoa, 1976). Some studies, moreover, indicate that the recovery of the children that do improve cannot be explained readily in terms of the knowledge gained by the mother. Neither have attempts to explain differences in recovery rates by reference to social or economic factors been notably successful. In general, however, the influence of nutrition education on the mother has been but little studied; likewise, other social influences that affect her behaviour have not received much attention.

The difficulties facing evaluative studies of such centres and of similar programmes are considerable. The education is commonly given to heterogeneous populations, whose food habits often vary. Moreover, whatever criteria of success are selected, these will inevitably be open to influences beyond that of the education: infections, for example, also have a deleterious effect on nutritional status. Furthermore, the selection of control groups is often extremely difficult. Neither nutrition education nor its evaluation is a simple and clear-cut matter, particularly under the circumstances prevailing in many developing countries. If we wish to gain insights into nutrition education - its functioning and reception among such populations - it will be necessary to study the process which intervenes between the educational input and the final outcome, the health status of the child. This means that we must consider not only nutritional status, but also the mother's understanding, attitudes, and beliefs, and also the impact of external variables. This approach to evaluation is heuristic rather than simply an assessment of results, and it is with this kind of evaluative research that this monograph is concerned.

Since, in this context, this was a new type of study, an exploratory approach was required. Indices to measure understanding and attitudes had to be developed and tested before any evaluation could be carried out. Constraints on time and money further limited the possibility of making a full comparison of N.R.C.s and alternative programmes. Such a project would have entailed a considerable disruption of these programmes, which were already well established, and would have created high expectations of the findings. Neither event was desired. Rather, a series of small-scale studies was carried out which did not make serious demands upon, or greatly interfere with, the daily operations at the centres.

We started by collecting general information on the different nutrition education programmes, aiming at improving the health of small children, that were operating in Uganda at the time. Most programmes were visited, and they are described at the end of Chapter 1. This first chapter, after a brief description of Uganda and its population, discusses some pertinent aspects of agriculture, food, and nutrition in the country. This chapter also reviews the incidence and immediate causes of childhood malnutrition and describes the various educational programmes. From these programmes we selected three for further study. These are (A) the inpatient, and (B) the outpatient, departments of the main nutrition rehabilitation centre in Uganda, situated in Kampala, and (C) an outpatient clinic at Luteete some 40 miles from the capital. Chapter 2 gives a more detailed description of these three clinics and of the evaluation that had previously been carried out. The problems confronting evaluative research in such settings are discussed in greater detail in Chapter 3.

Chapter 4 describes the methods of evaluation that were subsequently employed at the three selected clinics. The study designs and the indicators used to assess changes are described (the development of the indicators is presented in detail in Appendix B). The results presented in Chapter 5 are analysed with respect to the viability of the evaluative methods and to the effectiveness of the teaching, and some findings are further explored in a second study. The results of this second study, which concentrated on attitudes, are reviewed in Chapter 6. In a third study (Chapter 7) first- and final-year students at teacher training colleges were interviewed with the same schedules as were used in Study 1. We felt that it was important to investigate the knowledge and attitudes of these students who will be teaching future generations of mothers and fathers.

Chapter 8 (Study 4) describes an investigation into the social factors that contribute to poor or good nutritional recovery, utilizing the extensive case records of the outpatient section of the central N.R.C. in Kampala. This is followed in Chapter 9 by a model which shows the place that nutrition education occupies within the constellation of social factors influencing the child's nutritional progress. Study 5 attempts to assess the relative importance of these various factors in an interview study carried out among mothers regularly attending the outpatient department. Finally, in Chapter 10, some general conclusions are drawn about nutrition education and its evaluation. In addition, certain recommendations are made regarding the actual programmes that were studied.

The present monograph first aims at being a contribution to methods in evaluative research. It not only indicates the complexity of such research in the case of nutrition education in developing countries but also demonstrates the intricacy of the methods required.

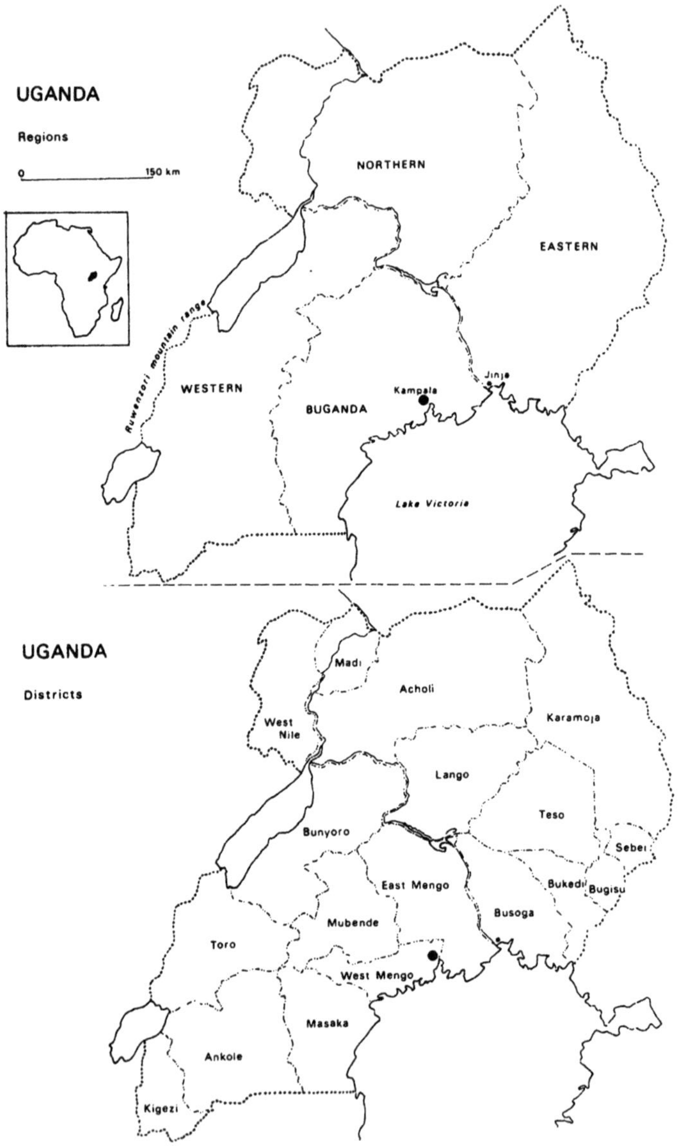

Figure 1. *Uganda: regions and districts*

1 Protein-Energy Malnutrition in Uganda

Uganda lies in the centre of Africa, to the north and west of Lake Victoria, the largest inland lake of Africa. Most of the country forms part of a high plateau and is well endowed with respect to climate and soil. Although situated on the equator, the high altitude and the presence of Lake Victoria produce a moderate climate in the south, while in the north temperatures are higher. The country is characterized by wooded savannahs and grasslands; and soils, in general, are fertile under the prevailing conditions.

Until recently[1] the country was divided into 4 administrative regions which were sub-divided into 18 districts (see map, Figure 1). At the time of the 1969 population census, the African population numbered 9½ million and it was exptected to reach 12 million in 1976. Bantu tribes form 60-70 per cent of the population and inhabit the Western region, the southern part of the Eastern region, and Buganda. The Northern region and the north of the Eastern region are inhabited by Nilo-Hamitic and Nilotic tribes, each of which represents around 15 per cent of the population. The largest individual ethnic group is the Baganda which lives in the central province, Buganda, where the capital, Kampala, is also situated. The vast majority of the people live in rural areas, and there are few sizeable towns. In 1969 Kampala had a population of 330 000 people while Jinja, the second largest town, had only 52 000 inhabitants. At that time only 7 per cent of the population lived in towns of more than 2000 inhabitants.

Among the population 19 per cent are 4 years of age or

younger, and 27 per cent are between 5 and 14 years old. By the time a woman reaches 45 years of age, she will on average have given birth to 7 children, but 12 out of every 100 babies die before they reach their first birthday. The natural population increase is estimated at 3 per cent per year.

Although the education level of the population compares favourably with that of other African countries, 62 per cent of the African population of over 4 years of age has never had any formal education: that is, 51 per cent of the men and 73 per cent of the women. For those who attended primary schools, education is generally limited to a few years.[2]

1.1 Agriculture, food, and nutrition

The Ugandan economy is dependent mainly upon the rural production sector, in particular upon agriculture, with 90 per cent of the population depending on farming for its livelihood (Uganda Government, 1972). The major cash crops are coffee and cotton. Cotton is grown mainly in the east and the north, whereas coffee is grown to the south in areas alongside Lake Victoria. Both cash crops are grown largely by individual farmers and their families on smallholdings where they also grow food crops for their own consumption (*Atlas of Uganda,* 1967).

The main food crop among the Bantu tribes in the south is matooke, a cooking banana, with sweet potatoes and cassava serving as alternative staple foods. Finger millet is the staple food of the Nilo-Hamitic tribes, while cassava is consumed primarily by the Nilotic tribes in the north, where sweet potatoes also serve to vary or supplement the staple diet. Legumes such as groundnuts, beans, and peas are grown in lesser quantities throughout the country but least in the northern region (*Atlas of Uganda,* 1967; McDowell, 1972). Meals usually consist of a staple food (bananas, cassava, sweet potatoes, millet) as the central dish, together with a small portion of relish which may consist of legumes, vegetables, or occasionally of animal products. The energy value (calories) and protein content of various foodstuffs per 100 grams of edible portion are presented in Table 1. As regards the staple foods, bananas and sweet potatoes are very low in both calories and protein content. Cassava flour contains equally little protein, although more calories; but when the cassava is eaten fresh, its calorie content is as low as that of sweet potatoes. Finger millet and rice are the most nutritious of the staple foods. The legumes provide far richer sources of nutrients in terms of both calories and proteins. Most vegetables are low in calories as well as in proteins. Where bananas, sweet potatoes, or cassava form the main component of the diet, an individual must consume large amounts of food to meet his nutritional requirements. It is evident that the legume relishes form an important source not only of proteins but also of calories. Research into local food practices has shown that small children often consume little of these relishes.

Table 1. *Nutrient content of various foodstuffs (per 100 grams of edible portion)*

	Calories	Proteins (grams)
Staple foods:		
bananas, cooking	100	1.5
sweet potato	166	1.3
cassava flour	350	1.8
finger millet meal	346	8.7
rice, polished	360	7.5
Legumes:		
groundnuts, shelled	577	27.1
beans, dry, mixed	330	19.5
cow peas	330	22.4
Vegetables:		
cabbage	23	1.5
onion	48	1.5
tomatoes	20	1.0

Source: Burgess and Burgess (1972).

Estimates by different authors suggest that for the country and the population as a whole, food availability and food requirements are fairly well balanced (Cleave, 1972; McDowell, 1972). Uganda is generally not regarded as threatened by food shortages (May and McLellan, 1970). McDowell (1972), however, by breaking down the overall figures, has shown that there exist considerable differences in food availability between the four regions of the country. The Eastern and Northern regions appear much better off than Buganda and the Western region, where the balance between requirements and availability seems to be at best precarious. Adult starvation, however, is rare in the country, with the exception of Karamoja district. In the rest of the country, adult malnutrition occurs only incidentally; and when it does occur, it seems to result from a breakdown of the traditional forms of care for the old and the infirm rather than from an actual shortage of food (Bennett and Stanfield, 1971). The vulnerable group of infants and young children, however, is in greater danger.

1.2 The prevalence of protein-energy malnutrition of early childhood

Protein-energy malnutrition of early childhood ranges from mild through moderate degrees, to the severe manifestations of kwashiorkor and marasmus. Kwashiorkor patients are generally characterized by oedema, muscle wasting, and severe apathy, while hair and skin changes also frequently occur. Marasmic patients are characterized primarily by extreme wasting, the child appearing to be of mere skin and bones. To complicate the picture, however, most malnourished children in Uganda exhibit mixed syndromes, whether severe, moderate or mild, that defy precise classification (Jelliffe and Stanfield, 1966). Throughout this monograph, the terms malnutrition, childhood malnutrition, and protein-energy malnutrition are used interchangeably. In accord with recent usage, the term protein-energy malnutrition is preferred to that of protein-calorie malnutrition.

Precise prevalence estimates of childhood malnutrition are difficult to obtain. Reliance on clinic records tends to give an underestimate because not all malnourished children are brought to a clinic, while the problems of defining malnutrition complicate the interpretation of survey data. Nevertheless, a number of studies over the years indicate a relatively high prevalence of malnutrition among young children in Uganda.

Burgess (1962,a,b,c,d,e) counted the total number of children under five years of age who suffered from kwashiorkor or marasmus and who were seen at dispensaries or admitted to hospitals in five districts in the Western and Eastern regions during the course of one year. This number of children was expressed as a percentage of the total number of children between eight months and five years of age living in each district (Dean and Burgess, 1962). These prevalence figures varies from 0.5 per cent to 1.3 per cent.[3]

Previous surveys by Gongora and McFie (1959) reported much higher incidence rates. These authors recorded the number of children under six years of age suffering from kwashiorkor or marasmus who were seen at selected dispensaries over an average period of eight weeks. This total was expressed as a percentage of the number of children attending the dispensaries during the same period. For nine districts in Eastern, Western, and Buganda region these percentages varied from 5 per cent to 17 per cent.[4]

Jelliffe and his co-workers carried out a series of surveys in selected villages in the Northern region. In West Nile (1962) all children under four years, in Acholi (1963) all children under five years, and in Karamoja (1964) all 'pre-school' children, living in these villages were examined. The point prevalence of severe malnutrition was 1.0-1.1 per cent in each of the three districts. Low body weight, however, was much more prevalent. In West Nile and Acholi districts, 6.6 and 4.3 per cent of the children suffered from third degree of malnutrition according to the Gomez classification based on weight for age. Many more children (75 and 63 per cent, respectively) were suffering from mild, i.e. first degree, malnutrition. A similar survey was carried out in Kigezi district in the Western region (Jelliffe *et al.*, 1961) and here 1.5 per cent of the children under four years suffered from severe malnutrition, while 43 per cent showed first degree of malnutrition.

Although the percentages of severe malnutrition reported in

these last surveys hover around 1 per cent, just as in Burgess's (1962,a,b,c,d,e) surveys, this is misleading. Jelliffe *et al.* recorded the children that suffered from severe malnutrition at one particular point in time, whereas Burgess's records covered one full year. Jelliffe's findings, therefore, point to a higher prevalence of severe malnutrition than the figures presented by Burgess. Thus, according to the most conservative (and probably under-) estimate, 1 per cent of the children under five years of age suffer from severe malnutrition each year, which in 1969 would have meant at least 18 000 children.

Among children with severe malnutrition who were admitted to hospitals in Uganda a mortality rate of around 20 per cent has been observed (Wharton, 1971). The mortality rate of untreated severe malnutrition is unknown but is likely to be much higher. The number of children who died from malnutrition in Uganda between 1960 and 1963 has been estimated at 5000 to 7000 each year (Wharton, 1971).

The cases of severe malnutrition, however, are only the tip of a veritable iceberg of less overt undernutrition. Recent insights into the evolution of malnutrition tend to view kwashiorkor and marasmus as resulting from the same long-term process (Rao, 1974). In the typical case in Uganda malnutrition starts after the first six months of life with growth failure. As this process continues the child becomes increasingly marasmic. This

> . . . progressive wasting of body tissues is a means of maintaining homoeostasis in the face of energy and protein deprivation. It seems probable, however, that adaptation may fail at any point during the wasting process, depending on several factors, such as the balance of energy and protein in the diet, the presence of concomitant infection, and so on. It may even be that the process of wasting eventually reaches a critical point (if the individual survives) at which no further adaptation is possible, and homoeostasis fails. (Hay, Whitehead and Spicer, 1975, p. 429.)

A more fundamental distinction can therefore be drawn between 'chronic undernutrition' and 'acute malnutrition'. Chronic undernutrition is indicated by the degree of wasting of body tissues and impairment of growth, whereas acute malnutrition is reflected by metabolic abnormalities. There are indications that the process of chronic undernutrition in the long run has more serious consequences than an episode of acute malnutrition, as demonstrated by Hoorweg and Stanfield (1976) for intellectual abilities.

Such chronic undernutrition among young children is widespread. The findings of Jelliffe *et al.* (1961, 1962, 1963, 1964) reported above indicate that at any one time 40 per cent or more of the children suffered from first degree malnutrition. The results of two biochemical tests among selected groups of children under four years of age in Buganda and Bukedi showed signs of malnutrition in 32-47 per cent of the cases, although the incidence of severe malnutrition was less than 1 per cent in both groups (Rutishauser and Whitehead, 1969). In fact, after reviewing the evidence Rutishauser concluded, 'it may be that nearly every child in Uganda goes through a phase of marginal malnutrition or delayed growth at some time during the first four years of life' (1971, p. 15).

1.3 The immediate causes of childhood malnutrition

The reasons for the prevalence of malnutrition among young children in Uganda are complex, but the immediate causative factors are well known. A vicious circle, in which poor nutrition leads to a decreased resistance against infections, which in turn lead to a poor nutritional status, lays the basis for acute malnutrition. In recent years the important role that infections play has been increasingly realized. Brown and Opio (1966), for example, found that 40 per cent of the children admitted with kwashiorkor to Mulago Hospital in Kampala also suffered from infections. Infections not only contribute to growth faltering and loss of weight but also interfere with certain metabolic processes (Frood, Whitehead, and Coward, 1971; Gordon, 1976).

The young child has a limited capacity to consume food and is in need of a diet which is relatively high in calories. At the same time he needs relatively more proteins than an adult to sustain growth. Provided that the mother has sufficient breast milk, the child usually fares well till the age of six months. After that age, breast milk alone is insufficient to meet the nutritional needs of the child. In many African societies supplementary feeding is traditionally introduced about this age and usually consists of portions of the adult diet. About the age of one year, or earlier if the mother becomes pregnant again, the child is weaned. The task then confronting the child is clearly illustrated in the following passage:

> The normal meal pattern is usually of a central dish of the staple which is eaten with savoury sauces made from legumes, green vegetables and, occasionally, meat or fish . . . Tough 'chewy' meat is favoured and fish is normally cooked whole with the bones. These practices restrict the availability of these foods to young children who cannot easily masticate the meat and who will not be given fish because of the presence of bones. In these circumstances the young children may receive only the liquid in which the meat, fish or legumes have been cooked. Some legumes, particularly beans, which are often cooked in their stews are indigestible so far as young children are concerned and may cause diarrhoea. Children are also expected to fend for themselves at a fairly early age. Immediately after weaning the child may be set down at the adult meal and, although, at the outset, may be fed with portions of the staple dipped into the sauce by the mother or older children, he will be expected to eat by himself very quickly. In these circumstances the child's diet is likely to consist mainly of the staple and as much of the sauce he can manage to mop up . . . In general the only concession towards special requirements for children's foods relates to texture since it is recognised that young children should have soft or smooth foods. All too often this can result in extensive use of starchy low-protein foods such as bananas, cassava or sweet potatoes and, in these cases, the bulky nature of the food can result in repletion of appetite before nutritional requirements are met. (McDowell, 1972, pp. 149–50.)

The dangers of such a low-calorie/low-protein diet are enhanced by the usual pattern of meals in most homes. The Padhola household described below may serve as an example of many other households in the country.

Meal patterns vary at different times of the year, since they are closely related to patterns of work. There is a tendency to have the same number of meals each day, namely a snack early in the morning and two main meals during the day, but the timing changes. Cultivating is started early in the morning. Before the adults leave the house they may drink tea or eat some of the cold food from the evening meal, but often they start without 'breakfast'. Cold food is thought to be bad for children, to upset their stomachs and make them ill, but nevertheless, it is they who usually eat the leftover food. After returning from the fields, the wife prepares the first main meal of the day. A main meal should consist of a staple and a relish, but sometimes only a staple is eaten with salt and water. When farm work continues late into the day, this may be the only meal that is eaten if preparation takes a long time. In this case, a snack may be eaten on returning from the fields while waiting for the meal. Alternatively the first meal may consist of some dish which is quick to prepare. When a second meal is prepared in the evening, after a late first meal, the younger children are often asleep before it is ready. (Sharman, 1972, p. 81.)

Dietary inadequacy and infections are the general reasons for the relatively low nutritional status of many Ugandan children. This in itself may be enough to cause growth retardation and even severe malnutrition in otherwise normal children living in ordinary circumstances. As will be described in more detail in Chapter 8, social factors also play a role although probably not an overriding one. However, in a number of cases, such factors as early weaning, marital instability, and poverty among immigrant groups may aggravate the condition of the child.

1.4 Nutrition education

Initially (i.e. through the 1950s) care was aimed mainly at the severe cases, in effect treating the symptoms rather than alleviating the underlying causes. It later became clear that the causes were not only medical, but that chronic malnutrition also resulted from a combination of agricultural, dietary, and child-rearing practices. This meant that after hospital treatment a child would often return to the same situation which had contributed to his initial condition. Attention was turned to the mother's role in modifying that situation - both as regards treatment and prevention. In Uganda the earliest attempts to change infant feeding habits by means of nutrition education originated in medical circles. Over the years, other avenues were opened up, utilizing community development workers, social services, schools, and even large industrial companies. The mass media were little used. In order to describe the background to the present studies, the next section summarizes the range of nutrition education schemes in Uganda in the early 1970s, at a time when the country was still functioning normally.

Medical services

The *paediatric wards* of hospitals did admit a large number of severe cases of malnutrition. Treatment in the wards was predominantly medical, and, given the shortages of staff, the educational potential in hospitals was usually small.

Health centres represent an intermediate stage between hospitals and dispensaries. In addition to the normal medical staff for clinical work, a health centre also employs various instructors. Health inspectors and health assistants are concerned with contagious diseases and sanitary improvement in the homes; assistant health visitors give health education. The latter are qualified nurses or midwives who have taken a course of one year at one of the two schools for health visitors at Entebbe and Mbarara. In all there were about 60 of these assistant health visitors working in rural health centres.[5] Their duties concerned the welfare of the whole family, but they were expected to pay special attention to maternal and child care by means of health teaching at child welfare clinics, antenatal clinics, women's clubs, etc. They encouraged mothers with small children to attend regularly the child welfare clinic, where children were examined and individual advice was given. They also paid home visits to families in a '*defined area*' usually consisting of between 50 and 100 families living near the health centre.

Some *dispensaries* reserved one day each week for a child clinic, where the medical assistant examined the child and gave advice on child health and nutrition. Alternative systems that combined the benefits of a dispensary near the home of the family with a concentrated educational effort were the Luteete Maternity Centre and the Pre-School Protection Programme.

The *Luteete Maternity Centre,* in a small village some 40 miles from Kampala, was run by midwives and social workers under the supervision of Mengo Hospital, Kampala, and had four beds for cases of malnutrition. A weekly children's clinic was held by a doctor and a senior nurse, and mothers with young children were advised to attend regularly. While the mothers waited to see the doctor, lectures and demonstrations on child-feeding were given. During the week a social worker visited families at their homes. The clinic provided services over a broad front and malnutrition was viewed as a social problem, not as an exclusively medical one.

The *Pre-School Protection Programme*[6] was a mobile child clinic operating from the district capital of Mbarara. Once every six weeks teams of medical assistants, nurses, and health educators visited remote places in Ankole district, to which mothers of young children from that area were summoned by the local chief. Although the main aim of the programme was immunization and treatment, attention was also paid to the nutritional status of the child. Weight charts were given to the mother for each child and explained to her. Once the mothers had attended the clinic the health educator gave a short talk on child nutrition to small groups of them.

The pivotal programme, however, in the field of nutrition education was that of *Mwanamugimu,* a nutrition rehabilitation centre founded in 1965 and situated in the grounds of Mulago Hospital in Kampala. Since its inception this unit had become increasingly important both as a general centre for nutrition education and as a model for other nutrition education schemes. The staff of the unit included nurses, health educators, a medical assistant, and various other personnel. It had an inpatient ward (both mother[7] and child were admitted) and an outpatient clinic, and it also provided accommodation for various other groups such as trainee nurses and trainee health educators. Through these latter groups it had a considerable influence on nutrition education elsewhere in the country.

The basic idea underlying the clinic was to achieve the cure of the malnourished child with a balanced diet which the mother was taught to prepare. Medical intervention was kept to a minimum, so that she learned through her own experience that malnutrition can be cured by adequate feeding.

A few mission hospitals had copied the Mwanamugimu model, albeit with certain alterations and on a smaller scale. The chief modification of the Mwanamugimu model as applied at St. Joseph's Hospital, Kitovu near Masaka, some 80 miles from Kampala, was the creation of close links with regional health centres. These centres referred cases to the hospital and co-operated in follow-up after the discharge of the patients.

Community development

A further kind of education took place through clubs and discussion groups organized by the Ministry of Culture and Community Development in rural areas. The Ministry employed some 90 Community Development Assistants who received part-time assistance from local club members who had attended courses at district training centres. At the time of our studies there were about 300 of these trained club members, while there were some 4000 clubs, each with 25-30 members. The Community Development Assistant usually started a club by contacting a chief and asking him to convene a group of women. The women elected a chairwoman and secretary and organized their own activities, often inviting outside speakers. Topics included health, child care, agriculture, home economics, and handicrafts. Membership was by co-optation without any official religious or educational bias, but there was a lower age limit of about 18 years. Selected members could go to training centres to receive further instruction in various topics, and some of these women went to Mwanamugimu to follow a course in nutrition (they were the women known as 'area cases', and are described in the next chapter). The aim was that certain club members should be trained in a particular subject, and could instruct other members as well as neighbours.

In urban and peri-urban areas, similar clubs were organized, albeit on a smaller scale and by private organizations, such as the Y.W.C.A., the Uganda Council of Women, and the Mothers' Union. The Y.W.C.A., for example, employed one full-time worker, trained in agriculture, home economics, and nutrition. She toured the regional centres of the association which were situated chiefly near towns, where she gave talks and demonstrations on food and cooking rather than the medical aspects of malnutrition.

Industrial approach

Some commercial companies provide medical care for their personnel, and some even give nutrition education to the wives of their employees. With industrial growth such schemes may become of more importance, but in Uganda this approach was still limited. One of the few examples was the Uganda Company which organized health and nutrition clubs on several of its tea estates (Young, 1972). These 'agriculture and nutrition' courses comprised lectures by a trained nutrition instructor (of which the company employed three) followed by discussions. The emphasis lay on practical farming and nutrition, but health, hygiene, and child care were also covered, together with instruction in handicrafts. These clubs started in 1965, expanded rapidly, and ultimately there were between 800 and 1000 members. According to the company the courses were extremely successful and raised the standards of health and nutrition to such an extent that by 1970 they were being reduced in frequency.

Social services

Since malnutrition tends to accompany adverse social circumstances, it is a problem often met by the limited number of social workers employed in Uganda. Nutrition education therefore necessarily became a part of their activities, although it was limited in content and coverage. Nevertheless, this was one of the few educational activities aimed at the urban poor. The Save the Children Fund, for example, employed caseworkers in the towns of Kampala, Mbale, Fort Portal, and Kabale. These workers not only gave advice on nutrition to problem families, but also distributed supplementary foods.

Schools

All of the previous programmes aim their education at adults. Yet, it is often argued that nutrition education would be most effective if aimed at the future generation of parents, who are now attending school. Under the former colonial administration, considerable attention was paid in primary schools to 'home economics', in which aspects of family health and subsistence were taught. After national independence, the emphasis in the curriculum was shifted towards academic subjects, and home economics as a separate subject was abandoned. The home economics teachers joined the ranks of the ordinary primary teachers. Instruction in health and nutrition has been scattered throughout the syllabus, and it has been left largely to the individual teacher to decide what he will cover and what not. Moreover, even in the training of primary school teachers themselves only limited attention was paid to health and nutrition. These subjects were only incidentally taught, it being left to the colleges to decide the extent to which they would cover them. It was only at a few well-equipped secondary schools, such as Gayaza High School (Ssebaduka and Goode, 1972), which provided courses in home economics that significant attention was paid to nutrition.

Commercial approach

At the time of our studies there was one unique, commercial, programme run by the Africa Basic Foods Company (Harrison, 1972). This company processed and marketed soya products, for which the soya beans were initially imported but were later locally grown. The products included flour, porridge, buns, butter, and roasted soya beans.

The firm employed some 30 workers, including a promotion and sales department and their activities included nutrition education. Potential customers were contacted with the help of the Ministry of Culture and Community Development through the village chiefs who gathered groups of men and women. A talk was given on malnutrition and the concepts of protein foods and a balanced diet, followed by a demonstration in which soya products were prepared. Printed instructions for preparation were handed out, and information was also given on how to grow soya. Soya products were then distributed at reduced prices, and a local store was stocked with the products. The company maintained connections with several other programmes which either promoted or actually used soya products themselves. Despite its basic commercial orientation, the profitability of the company was minimal and losses were covered from outside sources.

From the programmes described in the last section we selected three in which to carry out the principal studies reported below. These were: the inpatient programme at Mwanamugimu, the nutrition rehabilitation centre in Kampala; the outpatient programme at the same centre; and the outpatient programme at Luteete Maternity Centre. The reasons for selecting these particular programmes are given below.

(a) In many countries, including Uganda, such medical services are considered the most important, and they incorporate many of the characteristics of the other programmes.

(b) An explicit request for evaluation had reached us from these clinics.

(c) Because of their size and method of operating they offered the possibility of studying relatively large groups of mothers and children.

(d) All three were situated in Buganda province and, thus, catered for populations of roughly similar ethnic composition. This population was composed mainly of Baganda but also had a large and variable group of immigrants both in the town and in the country.

(e) They were similar in certain characteristics yet differed in other important aspects. Mwanamugimu was an urban clinic for malnourished children drawn from a crowded and varied area. Luteete Clinic was situated in a rural area and catered for all young children, malnourished or healthy. At the same time a social worker helped to maintain strong ties with the homes of these families, ties which were lacking at Mwanamugimu. And yet, despite these contrasts, the content of teaching was very similar. In the next chapter these clinics will be described in more detail.

2 Mwanamugimu and Luteete Clinics

In Chapter 1 the nutrition rehabilitation centre in Kampala was identified as the most important setting for nutrition education in Uganda. This chapter describes the development of this unit, and reviews the evaluation that had been carried out up to 1970. Next, the Luteete family health centre is described with the basic evaluative material that had been collected there.

2.1 Mwanamugimu

In many developing countries 'nutrition rehabilitation centres'[8] have been established (F.A.O./W.H.O., 1966; Beghin, 1970; Beaudry-Darismé and Latham, 1973). Mwanamugimu was the first of its kind in Uganda when it was founded in 1965. Although there is considerable variation in the manner of operation of such centres in different countries, they share certain defining characteristics. These include that (a) they are intended for selected undernourished or malnourished children; (b) they operate primarily through teaching the mother how best to feed, and thereby rehabilitate, her child; (c) they operate at a low-cost, low-technology level, commonly as residential centres or day-care centres where mothers and children attend daily for several hours; and (d) they aim at extending their teaching into the community (Bengoa, 1964, 1967; Beghin, 1970; Beaudry-Darismé and Latham, 1973). Mwanamugimu[9] well exemplified these characteristics.

When it was founded, the clinic was intended to serve the urban population of Kampala and the rural inhabitants within a radius of roughly 20 miles, some 800 000 people altogether. Schneideman, Bennett, and Rutishauser (1971) estimated that about 13 per cent of this population would be in the age group of 9 months to 4 years, that is 104 000 children. They also estimated that in this area at any one time, some 3000 of these children might actually have frank kwashiorkor and that a further 30 000 would show evidence of mild protein-energy malnutrition.

Since the centre served such a wide area, the notion of an inpatient (IP) section was supplemented, not with a day-care centre, but with an outpatient (OP) department where mothers and children did not attend daily but received less intensive ambulant care. There were 20 inpatient beds, while the outpatient clinic typically catered for about 40 cases (new and repeat visits) each day. In 1966 the unit registered 1600 new cases and 8300 visits in all. From the outset, the great majority of the staff of about 20 were local Ugandan personnel, and during the period of the present studies the doctor in charge was the only European. The buildings were adapted from old, single-storey hospital wards, situated on Mulago hill on the outskirts of Kampala. Mothers and children were referred here from many other clinics in the catchment area and from the main hospital nearby.

Outpatients (OP)

Mother and child were received in a large waiting room, where their arrival was recorded by a clerk. Mothers attending for the first time were given a weight chart on which medical notes and details of the child's progress were recorded at each successive visit. These charts were kept by the mother, while at first the clinic also kept an extensive set of notes on each case (see Table 26, p. 97). As from 1971, the full notes were kept only for inpatients and for certain outpatients for whom special surveillance was considered necessary. Where a child was acutely ill, the registration clerk sent the mother directly to the inpatient clinic.

Next the children were weighed and their weights recorded on their charts. The women then waited in a group, in the section of the outpatient clinic used for the teaching. In comparison with the queues waiting outside a typical African hospital clinic, the setting was rather pleasant. The walls were decorated with educational posters and photographs depicting the progress made by malnourished children, with slogans which emphasized that the condition can be cured by correct feeding.

Around 10.30 a.m. the health educator gave a talk on selected aspects of malnutrition. The actual topics varied from day to day and are summarized in Table 2. Occasionally the health educator might select a mother whose child had made particularly good progress to explain to the rest of the group how she had applied the teaching to her own situation. The talk was commonly followed by a demonstration on how best to prepare a meal that would contain an adequate amount of protein for a young child. The emphasis of the teaching lay on preparing the protein component (e.g. meat, fish, beans, groundnuts) in a fashion which a weanling child can eat, and on mixing the protein foods with the starchy staple food. The mothers were also taught to serve the child's food in a separate bowl, rather than having him eat with the adults out of the communal dish.

Once the teaching session was over the children were examined individually in a separate room by a medical assistant who reviewed their progress. He selected from the new cases (and, occasionally, from those reattending) those children who would most benefit from admission to the inpatient ward. During the first year that the clinic was in operation, 8 per cent of the first visitors were selected for inpatient treatment, while a further 4 per cent were referred to Mulago Hospital for more intensive care. A child was selected for inpatient care generally if he was severely malnourished, especially if the mother lived far away and would find attendance at the outpatient clinic difficult. Cases with serious social or economic problems which would limit progress at the OP clinic were also admitted.

When necessary, a mother was also seen by the social worker to discuss in detail the problems she had in caring for the child; this was the main chance for individual counselling. Funds and transport were available in order that the social worker might pay visits to the homes of certain patients, and such visits were arranged during these interviews. Following these interviews, and

Table 2. *The content of the education at Mwanamugimu nutrition rehabilitation centre*

The instruction in both outpatient and inpatient clinics covers the following basic issues:

1. *Malnutrition:* Recognition, causes, prevention and cure, the importance of weighing children.

2. *Diet and child health*
   Pregnancy: Diet, weaning.
   Breast feeding: Duration, supplementation, dangers of weaning, criteria for successful feeding.
   Food preparation: The importance of vegetable and animal protein foods, the amounts of foods required by the child, the importance of boiling water and milk, child's meal should be prepared and served separately, need for varied diet, timing of meals, special recipes for the child.

3. *The use of certain special foods*
   Dried milk powders: Preparation, hygiene, dangers of their use.
   Sugar: Amounts required, how to include in the child's diet.

4. *Kitchen hygiene:* The centre has a demonstration kitchen, built of traditional materials but following a slightly improved design, including more adequate food storage facilities.

5. *Immunization and child welfare:* Importance of immunization; drug treatments in general.

6. *Food production:* The centre has a demonstration garden, in which several of the recommended varieties of vegetables are grown; rabbits and poultry are also kept for demonstration purposes.

As well as the above topics, the inpatients receive instruction on additional topics, including:

Table 2 (continued)

7. *Teaching methods:* The mothers are instructed in teaching methods, so that they can pass on to other women in their home areas what they have learned at the clinic.

8. *Finance:* Distribution of money and food priorities; the use of markets; additional sources of income for the family.

9. *Diseases:* Recognition and management of a variety of common childhood diseases (measles, malaria, diarrhoea, intestinal worms, skin infections).

10. *Additional medical information:* Obstetrics, family planning, lactation, common accidents to children.

continuing into the afternoon, small groups of mothers were taken to different parts of the clinic grounds where they received practical instruction on various topics. These included the techniques of growing the recommended foods (beans, groundnuts, and other vegetables), keeping rabbits and chickens, methods of cooking, and hygiene. For these purposes vegetables were grown in a demonstration garden and chickens were kept in a run. There was a demonstration kitchen and latrine, both built cheaply of local materials, but each representing improvements on traditional designs. For a small payment the mother could buy lunch for her child, prepared in the same manner as in the morning demonstration. No food supplementation was given, an exception being the provision of packets of dried skim milk, if available, to very poor mothers, chiefly those coming from the urban areas. The products of the Africa Basic Foods Company (chiefly soya beans and soya flour) were, however, sold at the clinic. Each mother was given a return appointment and left at about 2.00 p.m. On leaving Mwanamugimu many women attended an immunization clinic nearby.

Inpatients (IP)

The inpatient section comprised two buildings: one which housed the staff offices, a day room, and the patients' sleeping quarters; the other building contained a lecture room and the kitchen area. On her referral from the OP clinic, the mother went to the IP ward, where the child was examined, usually by the doctor. At this point children with very severe malnutrition, or those whose condition was seriously complicated by additional infections, were referred to the main hospital.

Whenever possible, medicines were not prescribed so as to demonstrate that the children could be cured by suitable feeding alone. To reinforce this point each mother herself cared for her child, under the guidance of the clinic staff. She herself cooked the food for her child. The kitchen consisted of several traditional cooking places (three stones), identical to the hearth in most homes except that the stones were raised off the ground. The use of crockery and general manner of food preparation was identical to that of most homes.

The direct intervention by the clinic staff was limited to the initial examination and to the daily case-conference and weighing of the child. These took place in the morning, and the mothers discussed with the staff what they had learned and the progress each child had made. An emphasis on group teaching and activities was a feature of the inpatient unit. A series of lectures was also given on the causes, cure, and prevention of malnutrition with extensive demonstrations of food preparation, covering the topics outlined in Table 2. With the emphasis on practical instruction, the women spent a large part of their time practising what they had learned about food preparation and about cultivation. By involving the mothers in caring for their children the clinic was also able to reduce the cost of its operation. Besides learning about nutrition, the inpatient mothers were also given instruction in child-care as well as in crafts such as weaving. On occasion, they also made visits to places of educational interest, such as the museum in town. On her discharge, the mother was given a 'diploma' with two photographs of herself and the child - one taken at admission, the other at discharge. Usually appointments were made for return visits to the OP clinic.

Area cases

A third group of women attending the clinic, known as 'area cases', provided the link between Mwanamugimu and the community development programme. The area cases were older women, who generally did *not* have a sick child, but who were selected by their village community to learn about child feeding at Mwanamugimu, in order to return home as nutrition educators. These women were generally club leaders, or women of high status, such as teachers, religious leaders, or wives of chiefs. Up to six places in the ward might be reserved for these women, who joined in the same activities as the inpatients. With the inpatients, they were taught how to teach and how to organize women's clubs in the villages, how to identify cases of kwashiorkor, and how to influence their neighbours towards better nutrition.

Once the area cases had returned home, the clinic staff were supposed to make periodic visits to discuss problems and to provide encouragement. Similar visits also had to be made to ex-inpatients to check on the child's progress, the standard of hygiene in the home, and the types of foods being grown. However, with only one vehicle available to cover such a large area this ideal was not fully realized and such visits were limited in number. By means of the network of area cases, the unit staff also gave occasional talks at schools, or to villagers in rural areas on aspects of nutrition. In all these activities the objectives were to restore malnourished children to normal health, to create an understanding of the nutritional requirements of the child, to modify food practices in the home, and to increase the awareness of the importance of these topics among community leaders.

Evaluation

The principal evaluative studies carried out at Mwanamugimu appeared in 1971 in a monograph of the *Journal of Tropical Pediatrics and Environmental Child Health.* Schneideman *et al.* (1971) compared the cost per case with the cost of hospital care, showing that Mwanamugimu was clearly cheaper, although the IP unit was more expensive than a small rural health centre. The authors also studied the success of nutritional recovery of 378 patients admitted during 12 months from February 1965. They reported that 34 per cent were recovering at a rate which might eventually eliminate their weight deficit, 44 per cent were making up their weight deficit to some extent, while the remaining 22 per cent were failing to recover when compared with standards for European children. These judgements were compared with clinical impressions, from which it appeared that the anthropometric data indicating poor recovery were not necessarily consistent with the clinical impressions. This already indicates some of the difficulties of judging a child's progress or recovery (see Appendix A). Schneideman *et al.* (1971) also reported that after attendance mothers had significantly higher scores on a knowledge questionnaire when compared with a control group. Finally, random follow-up visits were made to the homes of patients who had been discharged. Many of the simpler recommendations of the clinic (for example using a special pot for boiling water and constructing a child's latrine) were being followed by a majority of the women, whereas those innovations requiring expenditure (building chicken runs and keeping rabbits) were in general not followed.

A subsequent study by Robinson (1971) reviewed the development of the clinic from 1967 to 1969. He reported on the number of patients attending (37 outpatients per day) and the number of appointments kept (82 per cent) and discussed the correlates of successful rehabilitation. This he did by comparing 55 children who had recovered well (based both on clinical impression and on weight-gains) with 32 who had failed to recover. The two groups were compared in several ways, according to tribe, birth order, evidence of family disturbance, and several other variables. The results showed remarkably little difference between the two groups and certainly did not suggest any clear explanation for the failure to recover. Robinson also interviewed 63 mothers, enquiring whether the methods of food preparation which were recommended by the clinic were being used. Visits were made to the homes of 39 of these women, and 11 families were classified as 'good', 11 as 'poor', and 17 as 'intermediate' in terms of how the child's food was being prepared. On the same occasion the nutritional status of 60 of their younger siblings was also examined, and 19 (32 per cent) were found to be undernourished, suggesting that the longer-term aims of the clinic were not realized. There was, however, no clear relationship between the questionnaire findings, the home visit assessment, and the child's nutritional status (Robinson, 1971).

The conclusions that may be drawn from these studies are that a majority of cases do make reasonable progress, but that there are a substantial minority of cases for whom the teaching is not fully successful. It also is not clear why this may be, nor which women are least likely to respond to the clinic care.

2.2 Luteete

From the early experience at Mwanamugimu, and based on the idea that a programme of community care might be more successful in ensuring good progress, a weekly young-child clinic was instituted at the Luteete maternity centre in 1966. It was designed as a broad-spectrum clinic, with maternal and child health (M.C.H.) services as the core activity but also providing general health education, nutritional rehabilitation, and malaria prophylaxis. The health education included much of the teaching given at Mwanamugimu. The intention when starting this centre was to develop methods of care which could be reproduced in other, rural dispensaries. Therefore, it did not rely on a highly trained staff or on sophisticated equipment; and members of the local community themselves helped to construct the clinic buildings. The centre also engaged in extension work, in both agriculture and preventive medicine, in the surrounding community. A demonstration farm was started, with livestock and a variety of crops. Stanfield, in his description of the centre, commented that 'medicine provided the motivation and agriculture the means . . . A wider approach to rural family welfare was necessary and this would need the integrated assistance of all extension services.' (1971, p. 69.)

The development of nutrition rehabilitation activities came later, in 1968, and represented an additional activity to the routine medical checks on the children. When a child visiting the clinic (for whatever reason) was found to be underweight, the mother was told to reattend on a different day. The child's card (which was similar to that given to every mother attending Mwanamugimu) was marked, and a duplicate card made to keep a check on these 'at risk' children. These special clinics took place one morning each week. Each child was weighed and examined by a nurse. There followed a teaching session, very similar in content and method to the teaching at Mwanamugimu.

> During each attendance at the 'at risk' clinic the assistant health visitor, often aided by mothers of recovering children, cooks a mixed meal for the children and during the first few visits may supply a small amount of supplementary food. Every two or three months all the record cards are checked by the doctor and the assistant health visitor together, and re-sorted. Some children can be discharged from the 'at risk' clinic to return when need be to the general clinic. (Stanfield, 1971, p. 70.)

During the rest of the week the social worker visited families at their homes.

A small inpatient rehabilitation unit was started at the same time. The food for these inpatients came in part from the demonstration farm but in part had to be provided by the mothers. The inpatient unit was not in continuous use, but could accommodate two mothers with their children when the need arose.

Stanfield (1971) compared the cost of running the nutrition rehabilitation section with that of Mwanamugimu, and found the costs at Luteete to be considerably less. He also analysed the weight-gains of the first children attending the 'at risk' nutrition clinic during 1968 and 1969. Using the method described by Schneideman *et al.* (see above), he showed that 28 out of the 42 outpatient cases (67 per cent) were recovering well enough to eliminate their weight deficit. This compared with Schneideman's figure of 34 per cent at Mwanamugimu. Of the former inpatients, 21 out of 24 (87 per cent) fell into the 'successful recovery' group. Only 9 (14 per cent) of all 66 cases were failing to make acceptable progress, judged from their weight gains.

Because most mothers live nearby they continue attending which made it possible to record the long-term progress of these cases. This was frequently impossible at Mwanamugimu as the mothers generally ceased to attend when the child had recovered. At Luteete they commonly returned to the clinic for other reasons. Stanfield (1971) outlined three grades of long-term growth of the children discharged from the 'at risk' clinic or from the inpatient unit, which were similar to Schneideman's three grades of recovery from malnutrition. Grade 1 included children growing as much as expected according to standards for European children, Grade 2 covered those putting on some weight, although less than expected by these standards; and Grade 3 included those who were failing to gain weight over the assessment period of at least three months following discharge. The progress of 126 cases (OP and IP) on whom data were available are presented in Table 3. Out of the 126 children examined, 80 (63 per cent) continued growing satisfactorily, but the growth patterns of the remaining 37 per cent fell into Grades 2 and 3, and were below normal. The initial good results achieved in the 'at risk' clinic are not so well maintained into the longer-term growth phase.

Table 3. *Long-term progress at Luteete (after Stanfield, 1971, p. 73)*

Grade	1	2	3	
Number of children	80	35	11	N=126
(Percentage)	(63%)	(28%)	(9%)	

This ends the description of the three clinics that were selected by us for further study. Before these studies are presented, we wish to comment in more general terms on what evaluation at such centres implies.

3 Evaluative Research

'The need to evaluate critically the actual effectiveness of existing nutrition education e.g. nature, educational methods, content, time involved and resources required' has been expressed repeatedly (W.H.O., 1974, p. 402). A variety of publications further comments on the need for evaluation of nutrition education programmes such as N.R.C.s (F.A.O./W.H.O., 1966; Latham, 1972).

The *nutritional progress* of children attending N.R.C.s[10] is usually estimated from anthropometric measurements (Schneideman *et al.,* 1971; Robinson, 1971; Berggren, 1971; Cook, 1971; Eisler, Ravines, and Ramirez, 1969; Beaudry-Darismé and Latham, 1973; review by Beghin and Viteri, 1973). Some of these reports also present information on the extent to which mothers improve their *knowledge,* as an 'intermediate outcome', causally prior to the child's nutritional progress. This type of study is summarized by Latham (1972) in an F.A.O. monograph on the planning and evaluation of applied nutrition programmes. In other studies 'efficiency' (as opposed to 'effectiveness') has been estimated, usually by comparing the costs of N.R.C.s with the costs of hospital care (Beaudry-Darismé and Latham, 1973; Beghin, 1970; Eisler *et al.,* 1969; Bengoa, 1967). Finally, some attempts have been made to assess the *long-term impact* of the teaching, in follow-up studies with the help of home visits some time after the discharge of the child from the clinic (Eisler *et al.,* 1969; Schneideman *et al.,* 1971; Berggren, 1971).

One consequence of the development of nutrition rehabilitation centres and other educational programmes has been to make their evaluation more complicated than that of the hospital care they replaced. Intensive hospital care for a malnourished child may be relatively simply assessed by measuring the rate of growth that is achieved. Where a child does not respond to the care, this may with reasonable certainty be attributed either to an unsuitable diet or to the presence of complicating infections. In the case of educational programmes, on the other hand, the educational input does not have a direct effect on the child's nutritional status, but has its effect primarily through the intermediary of his mother's changing knowledge and behaviour. Here the diagnosis as to why a programme may not be succeeding if a proportion of the children do not recover is less straightforward. It might, for example, be due to an unsuitable teaching content or to poor teaching methods. Alternatively, the content may have been well expressed but not accepted; or, although accepted, the teaching may not have been applied by the possibly overworked mother. Here, the fact that children are not recovering adequately is not enough to indict the centre, and an analysis of the failure would also require information on these intermediate stages. Even where a programme is generally successful in terms of health improvement, there are usually a minority of cases who do not make good progress, while it is uncertain whether those recovering have made the best possible progress.

Writers on evaluation have distinguished several levels at which measurements may be applied. For example, Suchman (1967) specifies, amongst others, three different categories of evaluation:

(a) *Assessment of effort,* by which is meant the activities of the service team, and which may be measured in terms of visits made, patients seen, or money spent.

(b) *Assessment of performance, or effect,* which refers to the results or improvements produced by the effort. At N.R.C.s, for example, effect is commonly measured by noting changes in the child's nutritional status. Alternative terms include 'end-results' and 'outcomes'.

(c) *Assessment of process,* which consists of the analysis of why and how the observed effect was achieved. This provides an explanatory framework which, according to Suchman, is particularly valuable when a programme is not functioning successfully. In our opinion it is also a necessary component in the evaluation of N.R.C.s and similar programmes that try to influence health by means of education. The assessment of process in this case would include the mother's knowledge, attitudes, and behaviour.

The functional model which is implied here may be summarized as follows. The education seeks to alter the mother's knowledge, attitudes, and behaviour, either directly or indirectly, and through this to influence the child's health. Indicators can measure effects at each of these stages. None of these indicators is more important than the others; instead each contributes to an understanding of the composite picture. However, each part of this process is also open to other influences, including social pressures, economic availability, and so forth. These extraneous influences should also be included in the study of the process through which the education influences the child's progress. Such evaluative research not only requires special expertise but also is extremely time-consuming, two reasons why it can not be expected from the clinic staff as part of their routine duties.

In practice, there are two main aspects of method to be considered at the start of any evaluative study. The first concerns the choice and development of indices. The second relates to the choice of an appropriate study design; that is, what groups should be studied and compared.

3.1 Indices for evaluation

Improvement in the child's health is, of course, the ultimate aim of nutrition education. Measures of the child's nutritional status, the final outcome, may take several forms, but those most commonly used are based on the child's weight. This is because the objectives of many programmes are formulated in terms of child weights and because weight data are collected relatively easily. Other anthropometric measures can also be used, notably the child's height. And, of course, there also exists the possibility of utilizing biochemical indices. We will reserve the term 'outcome' to refer to indices of nutritional status.

But, as we have explained, the child's health is only one

criterion, and the most severe, by which the education may be evaluated. We advocate the use of 'process' indices in diagnosing the strengths and weaknesses of health education programmes in general, and nutrition education programmes in particular. Such process indicators should, in the first instance, cover the mother's knowledge, attitudes, and behaviour. In fact, several authors have studied the knowledge gains of mothers attending N.R.C.s but have found that the child's recovery is not readily explained in these terms (Robinson, 1971; Schneideman *et al.*, 1971). This finding is in keeping with evidence from behavioural research that the association of knowledge - and, for that matter, attitudes - with subsequent behaviour is weak. For that reason the net of evaluative research should be cast even wider to include also the role played by the social environment to which mother and child belong. In that way progress or lack of progress may be more fully explained. Some studies have indeed examined the social context within which the mother must apply the teaching (Robinson, 1971).

Having argued the need for studying the process whereby the intervention affects the child's recovery, in practice this is no easy matter. Instruments have to be developed which are reliable and valid or whose quality in this respect is at least known (of course, this applies equally to outcome indices). The first of our studies therefore concentrated on developing knowledge, attitude, and recovery measures. Indices of behaviour were not included because we lacked the resources to pay visits to the homes to make the necessary observations. A full description of the indices and their development is given in Chapter 4 (pp. 57 ff.) and in Appendices A and B (pp. 127 ff.).

3.2 Research designs in evaluation

Whatever the nature of the indices, the quality of the evaluation will depend equally on the research designs, that is, on the selection of the groups that are compared. Although it may be quite possible to draw a neat model for evaluation of, for example, N.R.C.s (Gordon and Scrimshaw, 1973), the application in field situations is always more difficult. In contrast to laboratory studies where the investigator often has considerable freedom to manipulate conditions and subjects at will, the evaluation of programmes that are already in operation faces many constraints. Although it is often quite possible to find solutions to such difficulties, these solutions are usually time- and labour-consuming. It then becomes a matter of choosing the right balance between effort and expense on the one hand and the quality of the data on the other. The following discussion will start from the generally accepted, pretest-posttest, design. It outlines the difficulties of applying this design in the practical circumstances of the three clinics which we studied. These difficulties are not unique and will be frequently encountered, be it elsewhere or with other types of programme.

The pretest-posttest control group design[11]

This design is basically a very simple one. A group of people are studied before they are exposed to a certain treatment (here, education) and again, afterwards, to observe any changes that have occurred. The inference to be made is that these changes result from the treatment. However, during this time period changes may also have occurred due to other causes, and they could falsely be attributed to the education. A control group is therefore employed which is not exposed to the treatment and which is studied at the same times as the first, experimental, group. Thus it can be observed whether any changes have occurred irrespective of the treatment and, if so, their magnitude can be measured. Further requirements are that the experimental and the control group are not inherently different and also that they do not react differently either to the education or to these extraneous influences. This leads to the design illustrated in Figure 2.

A sample 'AA' is selected from the population and randomly divided into experimental and control groups. Measurements made at 'time 1' compare the groups on the dependent variables. Subsequently the two groups are kept separate, the experimental group receiving education, while the control group does not. Finally measurements are taken at 'time 2'. The possibilities of

Figure 2 *Pretest-posttest control group design*

		time 1	teaching	time 2
population AA	Experimental group	0	X	0
	Control group	0		0

0 = observation or measurement;
X = the education which is being evaluated

realizing this ideal in field studies in general, but with our programmes in particular, are remote. Where a programme is already in operation the possibilities for controlling conditions and subjects are seriously curtailed. This threatens the application of the pretest-posttest design in several ways.

Consider first the requirement of studying the experimental group before and after the education. Because of the nature of the teaching, results cannot be expected in a short time, but only after an extended educational period. This is particularly true of outpatients, of whom it is difficult to keep track over a long series of irregular visits. Because reattendance is decided largely by the mother herself, it is extremely hard to ensure a regular lapse of time between the 'before' and 'after' measurements. Furthermore, certain cases simply do not make a specified number of visits but stop attending early. Two solutions are possible: to have someone waiting at the clinic permanently to interview the reattendants as and when they arrive, or to make home visits. Both methods are time-consuming and are limited by the fact that, for other good reasons, the routine records kept at these programmes are often minimal. Moreover, the first alternative does not solve the problem of irregular time-spans between interviews. As regards home visits it is usually very difficult to record addresses in such a way that the home can later be found. This is particularly so for rural areas.

The second obstacle in realizing the 'ideal' design lies in

choosing a control group. Selecting such a group from a population outside the programme runs counter to the requirement that control and experimental groups be selected from the same population. The children who suffer from malnutrition are arguably a selected group. It is possible that their mothers are characterized by poverty, lack of nutritional knowledge, or adverse attitudes, and that these may have contributed to causing the malnutrition. The alternative solution, of selecting a control group which does not receive any teaching, from among those seeking care at the clinic, poses ethical problems. The women have often spent money on travelling a long distance in the expectation of treatment, which alone makes it impossible to withhold it. Green and Figá-Talamanca (1974) have suggested that in some cases treatment may be deferred for the controls, rather than omitted. This is impracticable in educational programmes such as the present ones, because of the extended treatment they provide, and also because of the often acute nature of the child's illness.

One requirement in the pretest-posttest design is that experimental and control groups be kept separate to reduce the possibility of mutual influence or 'contamination'. This is especially relevant in education where the teaching could easily be communicated between the groups. While, in theory, this may be avoided by physical separation of the groups, this is no easy matter; and the irregular reattendances of the mothers increase the likelihood of such contamination. At the clinics that we had selected for study, such separation would at least have required a serious (if not near-complete) revision of existing procedure and was therefore not feasible.

This discussion leaves us with the conclusion that the application of the pretest-posttest design is often not possible in action research settings and was certainly not feasible at the programmes that we were dealing with. It is very difficult to interview the same women before and after the teaching. It has also been argued that an external control group is inadequate and that a control group must be selected from those attending the clinic, but that treatment cannot be withheld.

The reactions to the difficulties of realizing the experimental model in circumstances which do not favour it have ranged from a virtual dogmatism (Elinson, 1967; Houston, 1972) to an active desire to fabricate the best compromise permitted by the circumstances (Rossi, 1972). In the latter case one of several alternative, but less rigorous, designs may be selected. Campbell and Stanley (1966) emphasize that there is no single appropriate design, especially in educational research; but that we are confronted with a choice between several, more or less acceptable, alternatives. Such alternative designs are reviewed in several sources (Campbell and Stanley, 1966; Weiss, 1972); here the discussion will concentrate on three of them.

Static-group comparison design

The first possibility which naively comes to mind, is simply to take a group of mothers who attend for the first time and to compare them with mothers who have already attended a number of times. This design is known as a static-group comparison (Campbell and Stanley, 1966), and it is a procedure with pitfalls. Some of these follow directly from the previous discussion, but one in particular must be mentioned: that of self-selection. The irregular attendance of outpatients is related to selective reattendance: some women, after attending once or twice do not return. These women may have certain characteristics which distinguish them from those who reattend regularly: for example, they may be those who live further away from the clinic, or are least interested in the teaching. They may also differ in knowledge, attitudes, or behaviour from the regular attenders. When this particular group ceases to reattend, the level of knowledge and attitudes of the remaining cases may differ from that of the original group simply because of the change in composition of the group.

The results of this self-selection cannot be distinguished from the results of the teaching when relying on a static-group design. Any differences observed between the two groups may genuinely result from the teaching, but may also result from this selection process. Weiss has emphasized that:

> the cogent feature of the quasi-experimental approach is . . . the realisation that it is not essential to guard against every possible source of error. The aim should be to control those sources of error likely to appear in a given situation. (1972, p. 72.)

Since the static-group comparison guards against too few sources of error, its use is generally not recommended. There are other designs which are more acceptable, in certain situations. Two of these were used in the following studies.

Experimental-group only design

In the previous discussion of the 'ideal' design, we have argued the necessity of using a control group to distinguish effects due to other causes. That applies particularly to outpatient programmes, where the education takes place over a long period of reattendances, and where, for example, seasonal variations in food availability may occur. Such extraneous influences are unlikely to occur among inpatients who are interviewed at admission and at discharge. Inpatients are largely isolated from the outside world for a period of two or three weeks, and it is unlikely that influences other than the total experience provided by the clinic are responsible for the changes occurring during that period. Therefore among inpatients when studying the same women at admission and at discharge, one can on certain occasions dispense with a control group. We have used this design on one occasion in study 2, Chapter 6.

Posttest-only control group design

An alternative design is that known as 'posttest-only'. This design differs from the pretest-posttest design in that it leaves out the pretest measures (Figure 3). Campbell and Stanley (1966) suggest that if enough trust is placed in the randomization procedure one can dispense with the comparison of the two groups at time 1. In that case, it may suffice to study two groups once each, one that has undergone treatment, one that has not. In the

Figure 3 *Posttest-only control group design*

			time 1	teaching	time 2
population	AA	Experimental group		X	0
		Control group			0

0 = observation or measurement;
X = the education which is being evaluated

present case this means a comparison of women that have attended for some time with women who attend for the first time. In fact, this design is somewhat similar to that of the static-group comparison, except that - and this is the crucial difference - care is taken that self-selection does not occur. Experimental and control groups must be randomly drawn from the same population. Campbell and Stanley (1966) go so far as to include this design among the few true experimental ones, although other authors (Weiss, 1972) consider it one of the quasi-experimental designs. The crucial requirement, of course, is to ensure that the two groups are drawn from the same population. How can this be achieved?

First it is necessary to observe whether selective reattendance does indeed occur, and to what factors this can be attributed. Once these factors are known, it becomes possible to select the control group and the experimental group in such a way that they do not differ in these characteristics. This can be achieved in several ways, for example by matching case for case, that is by finding for each case in the experimental group a case in the control group equal on the selected characteristics. There are, however, serious complications inherent in this procedure. The self-selection effect can also be countered by limiting the study population in such a way as to include only those who do reattend. This omits from the control group those who are likely not to reattend, on the basis of the factors causing the selection.[12] For one thing, this design rules out the influence of seasonal variations. Admittedly it limits the evaluation to those cases who reattend a number of times, while no attention is paid to those cases who drop away. However, it seems fair enough to restrict the evaluation of the education to those cases who have actually followed it.

None of these procedures is completely satisfactory, because the possibility can never be ruled out completely that other selecting principles are also operating (and on this the discussion usually concentrates). Nevertheless, they offer more practicable designs for the evaluation of programmes such as the clinics we wished to study. Study 1 described in the next chapter utilizes the posttest-only design on all three occasions.

4 Three Nutrition Programmes

First Studies: Method

4.1 Design

For the various reasons discussed in the previous chapter, the 'posttest-only' design was utilized at all three clinics. Women were randomly selected from those first attending Mwanamugimu and Luteete outpatient (OP) clinics and from those being admitted to the Mwanamugimu inpatient (IP) clinic, and were interviewed. From among these women three control groups were later selected in the manner described below.

The experimental groups, the groups of women who had been exposed to the teaching, were randomly selected from the regular attenders. At the IP clinic, regular attenders were women who had completed the course. Regular attenders at the OP clinics were regarded as those women who had attended between six and ten times at Mwanamugimu, and who had attended five times or more at Luteete. Since most cases attend Mwanamugimu only a certain number of times, the upper limit of ten visits was imposed. (The average number of visits reported by Robinson (1971) was 5.9.) At Luteete the mothers often attend for years, so no upper limit was imposed on the number of visits. At Luteete the regular attenders include both mothers who had and mothers who had not received extra nutrition teaching. The sparse record-keeping relating to the extra teaching did not allow us to differentiate between these two groups. The difference between five visits at Luteete and six visits at Mwanamugimu as starting points is accidental.

As explained in the previous chapter, using the 'posttest-only' design under the circumstances at these clinics we had to guard against any differences arising through self-selection. Table 4 presents information for the random groups of first and regular attenders on five factors that might possibly lead to such selection and that at the same time might also be related to knowledge, attitudes, behaviour, or health of the child. These are the sex of the attendant accompanying the child (they were all women), whether Baganda or not, her education, relation to the child, and the distance she lives away from the clinic. Among the Mwanamugimu IP there was no indication of any selection throughout the course and it is true that very few mothers did leave prematurely. Among the outpatients it was evident that distance was the influential variable. Other authors have also reported that the one variable which seems to affect regular attendance at health services is the distance people have to travel (Moffat, 1969; Robinson, 1971).

A closer look at the regular attenders at Luteete revealed that none of them came from further away than 15 miles, but that several first attenders lived further away. These usually were mothers not living in the Luteete area but staying with relatives

Table 4. *Study 1. Characteristics of first and regular attenders at Mwanamugimu and Luteete*

	Mwanamugimu IP		Mwanamugimu OP		Luteete OP	
Groups*	1	2	1	2	1	2
Sex attendant: female (percentage)	100	100	100	100	100	100
Tribe: Ganda (percentage)	41	44	69	60	64	64
Attendant: mother (percentage)	79	78	84	96	94	96
Education: years of schooling (mean)	3.0	1.6	2.8	2.8	3.1	3.2
Distance to clinic: miles (median)	40	50	13.0	3.0**	5.5	3.1**
	N=29	N=27	N=32	N=25	N=36	N = 47

* 1 = First attenders; 2 = Regular attenders

** χ^2 p<.001

for a short period; such cases are unlikely to return regularly. It was therefore decided to omit from the group of first attenders the 12 cases coming from more than 15 miles away and to employ the remaining cases as a control group. Among the Mwanamugimu outpatients we found that only three of the regular attenders came from further away than 15 miles. Again a control group was selected, composed of those first attenders who lived less than 15 miles away. Three cases who came from further away were, however, retained to match on distance and tribal background the three regular attenders who lived far away. The IP groups were retained without any changes in their composition. The characteristics of the resulting experimental and control groups were then very similar (Table 5). The groups included only women and at each clinic the respective groups were very much alike in tribal composition, while the average education hovered around three years. Some 80 per cent or more of the cases were brought in by their mothers. Of course the groups no longer differed in the distance that the women lived from the clinics. As far as the regular attenders at the two OP clinics were concerned, two-thirds of them were Baganda, each lived a median distance away of 3 miles, had attended school for three years on average,

Table 5. *Study 1. Characteristics of experimental and control groups after omission of selected cases*

	Mwanamugimu IP		Mwanamugimu OP		Luteete OP	
Groups*	1	2	1	2	1	2
Sex attendant: female (percentage)	100	100	100	100	100	100
Tribe: Ganda (percentage)	41	44	63	60	67	64
Attendant: mother (percentage)	79	78	79	96	96	96
Education: years of schooling (mean)	3.0	1.6	2.9	2.8	2.9	3.2
Distance to clinic: miles (median)	40	50	3.3	3.0	3.5	3.1
	N=29	N=27	N=19	N=25	N=24	N=47

* 1 = Control groups; 2 = Experimental groups

and usually was the mother of the child. The Mwanamugimu IP group differed in that relatively fewer Baganda were admitted, and that many cases lived quite far from the clinic.

4.2 Indicators

As outlined above, this study concentrates on changes in knowledge, attitudes, and nutritional status. Since it could be expected that only a small proportion of the women attending the clinic would be able to read and write sufficiently to complete written forms, all material was collected verbally. This imposed a number of limitations. Verbal interviewing takes a considerable amount of time in itself and also has to be done individually. In all, it was deemed necessary to keep interviews down to less than 30 minutes. In verbal interviewing it also becomes necessary to use rather simple sentences since subtleties of phrasing tend to get lost. Furthermore, the number of answer categories becomes limited: a respondent cannot be expected to use a 7- or 9-point scale without pen and paper or other visual aids. Uneducated people tend anyhow to use relatively few answer categories. Although the women in general understood the questions quite well they usually preferred answers such as 'yes' and 'no', without finer differentiation. After considerable pilot testing we finally selected two knowledge scales, on disease and foods, and two attitude measures, the semantic differential and a paired comparison scale. The weights of the children which were recorded routinely at the clinic are used as outcome indices. The development of all indicators is described in detail in Appendices A and B; what follows below forms only a brief description.

Nutritional status

Two indicators of nutritional status are used. The first is a static measure, the child's weight expressed as a percentage of the weight expected for his age, utilizing the standards collected by Jelliffe (1966). The second is a measure of recovery rate over time based on increase in weight, which is described in Appendix A.

Table 6. *Knowledge scales*

A. Disease

(-) Imagine that you and your friend both have 2-year-old children but your friend's child stays smaller than yours. Should she be worried or does this not matter?
Correct answer: should worry.

(-) Can you give any reasons why your friend's child might stay smaller than your own child?
Correct answer: any reference to feeding.

(-) This is a picture of a child whose legs and feet are swollen, its hair is brown and it is miserable. What disease do you think this child is suffering from?
Correct answer: Malnutrition, kwashiorkor or any of the local names.

(-) What causes this disease? Once mention of feeding was made the question continued:

Did this child receive too little of the staple food or did it not get enough of the sauce?
Correct answer: sauce.

B. Food

(-) Is .... a body-building food?*	*Correct answer:*
milk	yes
matooke	no
English potatoes	no
paw-paw	no

* body-building food is the local concept used in the teaching to denote food with a relatively high protein content

Knowledge

From twenty questions included in the original questionnaire, eight were finally retained, forming two sub-scales. The first consists of four questions concerned with the recognition of malnutrition and knowledge of its causes. The second is composed of questions about the food value of four different foods (Table 6). The score of both indices may vary between 0 and 4, and they will be referred to as *Disease (knowledge)* and *Food (knowledge)*, respectively (see Appendix B.1). It is expected that with education scores will increase.

Attitudes: semantic differential

The semantic differential is a rating method developed by Osgood and his associates (Osgood, Suci, and Tannenbaum, 1957) and consists of a number of scales, each composed of two opposite adjectives such as good-bad, hard-soft, fast-slow. Subjects are asked to rate a concept on each of these scales. Osgood reported that in judging concepts people consider mainly three aspects which he termed 'evaluation', 'potency', and 'activity'. Later research has not clearly confirmed the existence of the latter two dimensions, but in a number of cross-cultural studies the evaluative factor consistently appeared as the most important component in judgement (Osgood, 1965). Material collected by the present authors among 200 Ganda secondary school students also produced a strong evaluative dimension and a less clear second dimension, here called dynamic.

In the present study this method was used to study people's conceptions of matooke (steamed plantain), the predominant staple food in this area. Respondents were asked to judge this concept against six 'evaluative' and four 'dynamic' wordpairs.

Evaluative wordpairs	good-bad
	happy-sad
	ideal-imperfect
	big-small
	important-unimportant
	rich-poor

Dynamic wordpairs	strong-weak
	brave-cowardly
	quick-slow
	active-passive.

Respondents were asked first to choose one of the two opposites or a neutral alternative (e.g. good, bad, or neither). When they chose one of the two opposites (e.g. good or bad) they were then asked for a further differentiation (e.g. very or not very good). This procedure effectively turns each judgement into a rating on a five-point scale. Scores for the two different groups of wordpairs were added so that two composite scores result: *Matooke Evaluative* with possible scores ranging from 0-24 (6×4), and *Matooke Dynamic* with possible scores from 0-16 (4×4). The more positive a respondent in his replies, the higher the score. The expectation is that with education the dynamic rating of matooke will fall, while the evaluative rating will show a smaller decline or none at all.

Attitudes: paired-comparison method

The semantic differential as used above gives information about people's attitudes towards one particular food, matooke, but a complementary aspect is that of actually selecting foods and meals for children. An index was drawn up that measured stated preferences. A forced choice paired-comparison scale was developed using six meals, three of which consisted of matooke (steamed plantain) combined with sauces that are low in protein and calorie content: plantain with bean soup, plantain with meat soup,[13] and plantain with cabbage (low-protein meals). The three other meals consisted of a far less popular staple but which was combined with three sauces that are high in protein as well as in calories: sweet potato with fish, sweet potato with beans, and sweet potato with meat (high-protein meals).

Mothers were asked to choose between two of these meals, the criterion of choice being implied in the phrasing of the question: *'which of these two meals would you prefer to give to a two-year-old child?'* In turn she was presented with all possible pairs (15 in all). The measure which is derived from these answers – further referred to as *high-protein meals* - is the number of times that a high-protein meal is preferred over a low-protein meal. There are nine such choices (3×3) and scores can vary from a minimum of 0 to a maximum of 9 (see further Appendix B.2). With education it is expected that the number of high-protein meals that are chosen will increase.

4.3 Procedure

As described in Chapter 2 outpatients arrive at Mwanamugimu, usually early in the morning, and are registered. The children are weighed and the mothers wait till about 10.30 when the teaching starts. As we considered it inadvisable to interview following a teaching session, all interviews were conducted before the teaching started on that particular morning. Patients newly admitted to the IP ward were interviewed on that or the next day. Inpatients being discharged were seen shortly before they left the clinic. At Luteete a similar procedure was in operation, with a teaching session half-way through the morning; but this teaching was often not concerned with nutrition, and on those occasions we interviewed throughout the whole morning.

The interviewing was always done by one of the authors, with the help of one of three experienced female interpreters, who translated questions into the local language, Luganda. The few women who did not understand this language were not included, but they were very few indeed. The interviews usually took place on a verandah outside the clinic at Mwanamugimu and under a tree at Luteete. These provided quiet places away from the crowd of crying children and chatting mothers. At Mwanamugimu at the conclusion of the interview we usually gave the child one of the soya buns sold at the clinic.

4.4 Summary

The first studies attempt to assess changes in knowledge and attitudes of the mothers of small children attending three clinics: the inpatient clinic at Mwanamugimu and the outpatient clinics at Luteete and Mwanamugimu. A posttest-only design was used on all three occasions, and care was taken to counter self-selection of attenders which might lead to spurious differences between experimental and control groups. Knowledge changes were assessed with the help of two scales, one concentrating on disease aspects, the second on the value of different foods in child feeding. Attitudes were studied by means of a paired-comparison scale asking for actual food preferences, and a semantic differential method which rated the evaluative and dynamic aspects of matooke, the widely preferred staple food.

5 Three Nutrition Programmes

First Studies: Results

Knowledge and attitude scores for the control groups at the different clinics are presented in Table 7. To remind the reader, these are the women being admitted to the IP clinic and the women who are beginning to attend the OP clinics and who are likely to attend at least 5 or 6 times. They are the people to whom

Table 7. *Study 1. Mean scores (and standard deviations) for control groups*

	Mwanamugimu IP	Mwanamugimu OP	Luteete OP
Disease knowledge	2.6 (1.1)	2.2 (1.2)	3.0 (1.3)
Food knowledge	1.5 (0.7)	1.8 (0.9)	2.0 (0.8)
High-protein meals	4.4 (2.8)	5.5 (2.2)	4.7 (2.2)
Matooke: Evaluative	19.1 (6.3)	16.2 (6.5)	17.1 (5.7)
Matooke: Dynamic	9.7 (4.2)	9.2 (5.4)	8.9 (4.4)
	N=29	N=19	N=24

the clinics mainly direct their activities, and a comparison across the groups will show whether, and to what extent, they differ. On the two knowledge scales the Luteete women on average score higher than the women attending at Mwanamugimu. This is understandable: Luteete is a general clinic with both malnourished and healthy children attending, while the cases at Mwanamugimu are all malnourished. The women attending Mwanamugimu appear indeed to be less knowledgeable both about the disease and about foods. There is also the suggestion that the staff at Mwanamugimu select for admission as inpatients those outpatients who already have a relatively good knowledge of the disease but are more ignorant about the value of foods. This is confirmed by the fewer choices of high-protein meals made by the inpatients and by their higher ratings of matooke. The Luteete first attenders are intermediate on these last three indicators, which suggests that the Mwanamugimu outpatients in general are not very different in their attitudes from the outpatients at Luteete, i.e. the general population with small children, although their knowledge is somewhat lower.

We now turn to the changes that were observed at each clinic.

5.1 Mwanamugimu inpatients

A comparison of the inpatient groups shows that all indicators change in the expected direction (Table 8). Both knowledge indicators show improvements, as do the choices for high-protein meals. The semantic differential demonstrates negative changes, in that the food matooke was judged slightly lower on both the evaluative and the dynamic dimensions. This accords well with the original expectations: the teaching comments on the low food value ('dynamism') of this staple, but avoids specifically denigrating the women's evaluative conceptions of it. However, where the women have thoroughly absorbed the teaching, their overall judgement ('evaluation') of the food is also likely to decrease. Differences between the two groups were tested with an analysis of variance which indicated significant differences on the knowledge questions, with the average number of high-protein meals showing a near significant difference. The same method for

Table 8. *Study 1. Mwanamugimu Inpatients: Differences between experimental and control groups (absolute and expressed as percentage of possible range of scores)*

Disease knowledge	0.8	(+20%)*
Food knowledge	1.2	(+30%)**
High-protein meals	1.2	(+13%)
Matooke: Evaluative	-0.5	(- 2%)
Matooke: Dynamic	-1.0	(- 6%)

Analysis of variance: * $p < .01$
** $p < .001$

testing the significance of differences was used in the sections below.

5.2 Mwanamugimu outpatients

The picture of changes at the outpatient clinic is less clear, and less easily comprehensible. As with the inpatient clinic, the two knowledge scales show a contrast between the two groups, but only that relating to the disease is significant. Consistent with the limited contrast in knowledge about foods, the difference in number of high-protein meals chosen is minimal. Surprisingly, however, the evaluative rating of matooke has risen in this group, while the dynamic rating has remained constant (Table 9). The increase in knowledge of malnutrition stands to reason: the teaching centres on the sick children, who are the mothers' basic reason for attending the clinic. It would appear, however, that at the outpatient clinic the staff are less successful than at the inpatient ward in teaching about foods and their values. In fact the results of the semantic differential scales suggest that (beyond simply not learning about food) the women actually interpret what was said in a contrary manner. These last results may, of course, represent chance error, as the differences are not significant; but since the food is used in many of the teaching demon-

Table 9. *Study 1. Mwanamugimu Outpatients: Differences between experimental and control groups (absolute and expressed as a percentage of possible range of scores)*

Disease knowledge	1.2	(+30%)*
Food knowledge	0.4	(+10%)
High-protein meals	0.2	(+ 2%)
Matooke: Evaluative	2.4	(+10%)
Matooke: Dynamic	0.1	(<+ 1%)

Analysis of variance: * $p < .001$

strations it is possible that the women infer that it is recommended.

Closer analysis reveals that the Ganda women, as expected, decrease their dynamic rating of matooke, but that they increase their evaluative rating (Table 10). The women from the other tribes, however, increase both ratings, evaluative as well as dynamic. Since the Ganda household forms the background of most of the teaching, the Baganda are perhaps better able to pick up at least part of the message. Perhaps the women from other tribes are not able to do so, and the very first thing which may strike them is an emphasis in the cooking demonstrations on matooke, which they themselves may use less. Interviews with the staff (see Section 5.5) shed some light on this curious finding, which is further explored in the next chapter.

Table 10. *Study 1. Mwanamugimu Outpatients: Differences between experimental and control groups by tribe (absolute and expressed as a percentage of possible range of scores)*

	Baganda	Other tribes
Matooke: Evaluative	+2.10(+ 9%)	+2.90(+12%)
Matooke: Dynamic	-1.67(-10%)	+2.99(+19%)

5.3 Luteete outpatients

The changes that occur at Luteete are all in the expected directions (Table 11). The knowledge scales show differences, although the difference observed on the disease scale is less than that found at the other two clinics. This is understandable given the emphasis in the teaching at Mwanamugimu that is laid on disease aspects, and on kwashiorkor in particular. The number of high-protein meals chosen also shows a significant contrast. As with the Mwanamugimu inpatients, the evaluation of matooke remains constant, while the dynamic rating drops slightly.

Table 11. *Study 1. Luteete Outpatients: Differences between experimental and control groups (absolute and expressed as a percentage of possible range of scores)*

Disease knowledge	0.1	(+ 3%)
Food knowledge	0.7	(+18%)*
High-protein meals	2.0	(+22%)*
Matooke: Evaluative	0.0	
Matooke: Dynamic	-1.2	(- 8%)

Analysis of variance: * $p < .001$

5.4 Comparison of mothers after exposure to the teaching at the different programmes

The knowledge and attitude scores for each of the experimental groups at the three clinics are presented in Table 12. To remind the reader, these are the women who have either completed an IP course or who have attended several times at one of the two OP clinics. How do they compare across the three programmes? The two Mwanamugimu groups are remarkably similar on all counts, much more so than they were before exposure. It was suggested

Table 12. *Study 1. Mean scores (and standard deviations) for experimental groups*

	Mwanamugimu IP	Mwanamugimu OP	Luteete OP
Disease knowledge	3.4 (0.8)	3.4 (0.7)	3.1 (1.1)
Food knowledge	2.7 (0.8)	2.2 (0.7)	2.7 (0.7)
High-protein meals	5.7 (2.9)	5.7 (2.9)	6.7 (2.1)
Matooke: Evaluative	18.7 (6.7)	18.5 (6.4)	17.1 (6.7)
Matooke: Dynamic	8.7 (4.5)	9.3 (4.6)	7.7 (4.4)
	N=27	N=25	N=47

early in this chapter that the inpatient clinic effectively selects the more ignorant but concerned mothers. Apparently, after the intensive teaching they are brought to a level of knowledge and attitudes similar to that of the outpatients after 6 to 10 less intensive sessions. Over all, the Luteete experimental group shows the highest scores except on the disease questions. Even so, on this indicator they still obtain 78 per cent of the maximum possible score. But it is on the attitude scales that the Luteete cases show the clearest contrast to the Mwanamugimu women.

5.5 The staff at Mwanamugimu

The staff at Mwanamugimu were also interviewed. Although the clinic has a stated policy that all staff personnel, from doctor to sweeper, should participate in the teaching, there is nevertheless a group of staff who are more involved in the teaching and advising than the rest, and these were interviewed. The knowledge

Table 13. *Study 1. Mean scores (and standard deviations) for Mwanamugimu staff (N=13)*

High-protein meals	8.1	(2.0)
Matooke: Evaluative	20.0	(3.3)
Matooke: Dynamic	10.4	(3.6)

questions, however, were not asked since they appeared rather easy for these trained workers and might have started the interviews on the wrong note. The interviews were therefore limited to the two attitude scales and the results are presented in Table 13.

The average number of choices for high-protein meals among the staff is considerably higher than among the control and experimental groups of mothers attending Mwanamugimu. Revealingly, however, the average ratings, evaluative and dynamic, of matooke are comparable to those of the mothers. In fact, the staff rated matooke more highly on both aspects. This, of course, sheds an interesting light on the finding that the outpatients increased their evaluation of matooke. The teaching given by the staff conveys information on the relative value of high-protein sauces over staples (as measured by the paired-comparison method), but it does little to bring about changes in the concept of matooke, the popular staple food, itself.

5.6 Nutritional status

Although the knowledge and attitude scales show consistent and revealing patterns, the question remains as to whether these correspond to similar patterns in the nutritional status of the children. This question can only be answered with the help of the two outpatient groups because the recovery of the children in the inpatient ward is closely monitored by the clinic staff and will therefore tend to show improvements independently of the results of the teaching. Table 14 shows the weight/weight-for-age ratio for the control[14] and experimental groups at the outpatient clinics. At both clinics there is an improvement in nutritional

Table 14. *Study 1. Average weight/weight-for-age (percentage) in different outpatient groups*

	Control	Experimental
Mwanamugimu	68.7 (N=17)	75.4 (N=23)
Luteete	77.2 (N= 9)	85.6 (N=42)

status with attendance at the clinic, while the children at Luteete are generally in a better condition than the children at Mwanamugimu, which is after all, a rehabilitation centre for malnourished children. Thus nutritional status shows variations similar to those observed in knowledge and attitudes over different groups. To what extent this is also the case for individuals remains to be shown. Since we are concerned with two different types of clinics - the one for recovery of malnourished children, the other for maintaining normal children in good health - different indicators of nutritional status have to be used for this analysis. As 'outcome' measure at Luteete, the weight/weight-for-age ratio is suitable, but at Mwanamugimu a nine-point recovery scale (see Appendix A) was used.

Table 15 presents Spearman rank correlations of the knowledge and attitude indicators with recovery and nutritional status at the two clinics. Not all the correlations are significant (which requires high coefficients among these small groups), yet they are all in the expected direction: positive for the knowledge scales and high-protein meals and negative for the two ratings. Multiple correlations in both cases are higher than .50 which means that some 25-30 per cent of the variance in nutritional status or recovery can be explained by variations in knowledge and attitudes.

Among the Mwanamugimu attendants the disease scale correlates poorly with recovery, perhaps because the children were already malnourished and making the mother aware of the disease does not help the child recover. It will be recalled that the main measured effect of the teaching here was, in fact, an increase

Table 15. *Study 1. Spearman rank correlations of knowledge and attitude scales with nutritional 'outcome' (outpatients)*

	Mwanamugimu: recovery	Luteete: weight for age
Disease knowledge	.17	.49
Food knowledge	.56	.09
High-protein meals	.25	.25
Matooke: Evaluative	-.13	-.08
Matooke: Dynamic	-.16	-.16
Multiple correlation	.60	.54
	N=21	N=42

in disease knowledge. Perhaps such knowledge may help in preventing relapses and in giving protection to younger siblings. In fact, at Luteete the mother's awareness of the disease and its causation appear to be important in protecting the child from it. That food knowledge does not correlate with nutritional status among this last group is unexpected, particularly since it does correlate with recovery among the outpatients at Mwanamugimu and because in both groups the number of high-protein meals correlated with the nutritional 'outcome'. The two ratings of matooke show low correlations and apparently are least related to nutritional status or recovery.

5.7 Conclusion

This study has, first of all, shown that it is possible successfully to use indicators other than nutritional status in the evaluation of nutrition education programmes. From the scales used in the present study the two ratings based on the semantic differential appear the least sensitive indicators. The tendency of these relatively uneducated respondents to use the endpoints of the scales has already been mentioned and has also been reported by Wober (1974). If they adhere to this, a change in attitudes will not show up unless it is so great that the respondent is willing to switch to the other end of a scale.[15] In the extreme, this means that she has to change her judgement from, for example, very good to very bad. Changes are usually not so dramatic. This leads to the conclusion that the semantic differential is probably of limited use in assessing such changes among uneducated populations, although the method can serve to provide descriptive meanings of a concept. In the present study the results obtained with the two knowledge scales and the paired-comparison method are more satisfactory. Particularly the results with the last instrument are encouraging because here is a measure consisting of questions outside the actual content of the teaching.

Employing such indicators may provide on occasion a fairer, and often a more refined, test of a particular programme. It has also been demonstrated that in this way insights can be gained which are not readily available using the more traditional means of evaluation. This is not to say that there is no need for 'outcome' indicators such as nutritional status. They are still valuable (at least when employed in conjunction with a sound design). Rather, we have demonstrated that other tools can also be utilized, which together with outcome indicators should provide a better understanding of the intervention.

6 A Closer Look at Food Preferences

The previous study found certain expected changes in knowledge and attitudes but left one with the vague suspicion that the mothers attending Mwanamugimu also learn to prefer certain staples which are often used at the clinic (see Section 5.2). The same results also suggested that among the Ganda mothers different processes may be at work than among the mothers from other tribes. The experience of that study had also given us the conviction that a paired-comparison type of instrument was best suited to look further into these attitude changes. This second study was carried out among inpatients and outpatients at Mwanamugimu.

6.1 Study 2: design

Among the outpatients a 'posttest-only' design was again used. In the first study we had found that distance was the main factor influencing reattendance; consequently the sample in this second study was also restricted to those mothers coming from a distance of 15 miles or less. Respondents were selected from those first attending and from those who had attended more than 6 times.[16] Table 16 shows that there are only small differences in the characteristics of the resulting control and experimental groups, none of which is statistically significant.

Among the inpatients an alternative design was employed, that of the 'experimental-group-only' (see Chapter 3), in which the

Table 16. *Study 2. Characteristics of inpatient and outpatient groups*

	Outpatients		Inpatients
Groups*	1	2	1,2
Sex attendant: female (percentage)	100	100	100
Tribe: Ganda (percentage)	46	48	52
Attendant: mother (percentage)	85	92	74
Education: years (mean)	2.6	3.0	2.5
Distance: mls (median)	3.1	3.8	12.0
	N=39	N=60	N=23

* 1 = Control groups; 2 = Experimental groups

same mothers were interviewed at admission and at discharge. The number of cases in this group was rather small because halfway through the collection of interviews a measles epidemic broke out (not uncommon at rehabilitation centres) and new cases were no longer admitted. The characteristics of this group are also shown in Table 16. It may also be noted that the groups are very similar to the groups used in Study 1 (Table 5, page 59).

6.2 Attitude measurement

The previous paired-comparison scale used two staple foods, plantain and sweet potato, in combination with six sauces. These two staple foods are also the ones most often used in cooking and demonstrations at the clinic. The present scale, comprising eight meals, includes two more staple foods, cassava and rice. This

Table 17. *Study 2. Meals included in paired-comparison schedule*

High-protein meals	*Low-protein meals*
(1) Plantain with meat	(5) Plantain with bean soup
(2) Sweet potato with beans	(6) Sweet potato with green leaves
(3) Cassava with groundnuts	(7) Cassava with cabbage
(4) Rice with fish	(8) Rice with meat soup

extended scale makes it possible to measure changes in preferences for sauces and for staple foods independently of each other.[17] The four staples are each presented twice, once in combination with a high-protein sauce, and once with a low-protein sauce (Table 17). Comparing the four high-protein meals (1-4) with the four low-protein meals (5-8) reveals the preferences for high- vs. low-protein sauces independently of the staple foods, as these are the same in the two groups of meals. (These choices can be found in the bottom left quadrants of the matrices in Table 19.) There are 16 (4×4) such comparisons, and the number of times a respondent chooses a high-protein meal over a low-protein meal gives the *protein index* with a possible range of from 0 to 16.

Subjects also make choices between the meals *within* each of the two different groups of meals. Preferences expressed on these occasions will be independent of the protein value of the two meals because they are both either high or low in this respect. These choices will reflect preferences for staples independently of the protein content of the meals. There are twelve such choices but our interest lies with the choices between a plantain or sweet potato meal, the meals used in cooking and demonstrations, on the one hand and a cassava or rice meal, on the other hand (meals 1,2 vs. 3,4 and meals 5,6 vs. 7,8). There are eight such choices and these are shown in the two smaller quadrants, above and beside the larger quadrants in Table 19. The *staple index* indicates the number of times that a plantain or sweet potato meal was preferred over a cassava or rice meal[18] and scores may vary from 0 to 8.

Table 18. *Study 2. Average number of choices for individual meals*

Groups*	Outpatients 1	Outpatients 2	Inpatients 1	Inpatients 2
(1) Plantain with meat	3.5	3.7	3.4	4.8
(2) Sweet potato with beans	4.1	5.0	4.0	5.9
(3) Cassava with groundnuts	3.2	3.5	2.7	2.7
(4) Rice with fish	3.8	3.8	4.2	2.9
(5) Plantain with bean soup	4.6	4.6	4.6	4.7
(6) Sweet potato with green leaves	3.9	3.6	4.3	4.5
(7) Cassava with cabbage	2.4	1.5	2.4	0.5
(8) Rice with meat soup	2.4	2.3	2.5	2.2
	N=39	N=60	N=23	N=23

* 1 = Control groups; 2 = Experimental groups

6.3 Results

Outpatients

Table 18 shows that among the control group of first-attending outpatients, preferences are evenly spread over high- and low-protein meals with an average number of 14.6 and 13.4 choices respectively. The meals with beans or bean soup are preferred, while cassava and rice when combined with low-protein sauces are least often chosen. Only two meals produce strong differences between the control and the experimental group: meal (2), sweet potato with beans, shows an increase, while meal (7), cassava with cabbage, shows a decrease. The first meal is a combination of one of the two staple foods used at the clinic with a high-protein sauce, the other a combination of low-protein sauce with a different staple food. This would confirm the existence of a combined shift towards high-protein sauces and 'clinic staples' were it not that the similar combinations (1) and (8) do not show this trend. The measure used here, the average number of choices for each meal, is, however, a figure that may both reveal and hide changes. It is, moreover, difficult to handle in statistical analysis because the total must always add up to 28, the actual number of choices.

The figures in Table 19A do not have such constraints since this matrix contains results for each of the 28 choices separately. Each cell presents the difference between the experimental and control groups in percentage of choices for that particular comparison of two meals. A *positive* figure indicates that the percentage of mothers choosing the meal on the top line is larger in the experimental group. Conversely, a negative figure indicates that the percentage of mothers choosing the meal on the top line is that much smaller in the experimental group (and, consequently, that much larger in the control group). A positive figure therefore reflects an increase in choices after education for the meal on the top line; a negative figure, a decrease in choices for that meal after education.

For the outpatients, 12 out of the 16 comparisons between the four high-protein meals and the four low-protein meals (which can be found in the large lower quadrant) show an increase in high-protein choices. However many of these are small, with only 4 between .10 and .20, while only 2 are statistically significant. These are no overwhelming changes.

The 8 figures in the two smaller quadrants, as explained previously, reflect changes occurring in staple preferences. Of these comparisons 6 are positive, implying an increase in choices for plantain and sweet potato, but the actual changes are even smaller than the previous ones, the largest being .12. The overall

Table 19. *Study 2. Preference matrix: Differences between experimental and control groups*

This matrix is obtained by subtracting the preference matrix of the control group from that of the experimental group. In these original tables each cell contained the percentage of choices obtained by the meal on the top line. The cells in the present table thus contain the change in percentage of choices for the meal in the top line. Positive figures indicate that preference for this meal was higher in the experimental group, negative figures that preference for this meal was lower in the experimental group. Positive figures therefore present an increase occurring with education, negative figures a decrease after education.

A. Outpatients (N=39 and N=60 respectively)

meals*	1	2	3	4	5	6	7	8
1	-							
2	-.06	-						
3	-.01	.07	-					
4	.09	.08	.09	-				
5	-.06	.14	-.01	-.04	-			
6	.05	.05	.06	.25**	.01	-		
7	.16	.39**	.10	.11	.03	-.04	-	
8	.03	.05	.09	-.07	.02	.12	-.15	-

B. Inpatients (N=23)

meals*	1	2	3	4	5	6	7	8
1	-							
2	-.05	-						
3	.31	-.05	-					
4	.39**	.61**	.22	-				
5	.13	.35**	-.09	-.27	-			
6	.13	.35**	-.09	-.09	-.05	-		
7	.26**	.39**	.17	.48**	.18	.22**	-	
8	.26	.13	.05	-.21	.09	.18	-.22	-

* 1 = plantain with meat
2 = sweet potato with beans
3 = cassava with groundnuts
4 = rice with fish
5 = plantain with bean soup
6 = sweet potato with green leaves
7 = cassava with cabbage
8 = rice with meat soup

**χ^2; $p < .05$

Table 20. *Study 2. Outpatients: Mean scores (and standard deviations) for protein index and staple index*

Groups*	1	2
Protein index	8.7 (2.4)	10.0** (2.3)
Staple index	5.1 (1.4)	5.5 (1.6)
	N=39	N=60

* 1 = Control groups; 2 = Experimental groups
** Analysis of variance; $p < .01$

figures for the *protein index* and the *staple index* (Table 20) show that the increase in preferences for high-protein sauces is statistically significant, but that there is no significant shift towards plantain and sweet potato. These results confirm the finding of Study 1 that there are changes in preferences towards high-protein sauces, but our suspicion about changes in staple food preferences is not confirmed by these figures.

Inpatients

The inpatients present a different picture. When newly admitted their ranking of the eight meals is similar to that of the outpatient control group, with only minor differences (Table 18). When interviewed at discharge from the ward, considerable changes have occurred in their expressed preferences. As explained previously comparing the average number of choices for the meals is apt to be confusing, and the changes that occur are more easily observed from Table 19B. From the large lower quadrant of this table it can be seen that on eleven occasions there is an increase in the number of choices of high-protein meals, and more importantly that several of these are quite high and significant. The fact, however, that five comparisons show a negative change, that is

Table 21. *Study 2. Preference matrix*: Differences between experimental and control groups, four comparisons combined (inpatients)*

		Plantain/Sweet potato with high-protein sauce	Cassava/Rice with high-protein sauce
	meals**	1,2	3,4
Plantain/Sweet potato with low-protein sauce	5 6	.24(I)	-.14(III)
Cassava/Rice with low-protein sauce	7 8	.26(II)	.12(IV)

* For an explanation how this table was obtained, see text and notes for Table 19.

** The individual meals corresponding with these numbers can be found in Table 17 and the footnote for Table 19.

a decrease in the number of choices of high-protein meals, must not be overlooked. In fact, an interesting pattern emerges when the meals are combined two by two according to their staple characteristics and protein value, as shown in Table 21. The figures in this table consist of the averages of the four corresponding changes in preferences already listed in table 19B. There are definite increases in choices for the high-protein meals as shown for those comparisons where there are no differences between the staple foods (cells I and IV respectively). Similarly there is an increase (cell II) for the meals that consist of a 'clinic staple' and a high-protein sauce when these are compared with meals consisting of cassava or rice together with a low-protein sauce. The most interesting figure is that in cell III, where 'clinic staples' combined with *low*-protein sauces are compared with cassava and rice combined with *high*-protein sauces. The negative figure means that when confronted with such a choice the inpatient mothers show a shift towards the plantain/sweet potato meals, despite the fact that these include low-protein sauces. These findings indicate that, when confronted with straightforward choices (e.g. a high- versus a low-protein meal with the same type of staple) the women follow the clinic teaching and choose the high-protein meal. But when presented with a conflicting choice between meals containing either a good sauce or else a staple used at the clinic, the experimental group chooses more according to the

Table 22. *Study 2. Inpatients: Mean scores (and standard deviations) for protein index and staple index*

Groups*	1	2
Protein index	8.3 (2.4)	10.2** (2.3)
Staple index	5.2 (1.6)	7.1** (1.0)
	N=23	N=23

* 1 = Control groups; 2 = Experimental groups
** Paired T-test; $p<.01$

Table 23. *Study 2. Mean scores on protein and staple index for Baganda and other tribes*

	Outpatients		Inpatients	
Groups*	1	2	1	2
Baganda				
Protein index	9.6	10.3	8.3	10.9***
Staple index	5.3	5.6	5.3	7.3***
	N=18	N=29	N=12	N=12
Others				
Protein index	7.8	9.7**	8.2	9.5***
Staple index	5.0	5.4	5.1	6.8***
	N=21	N=31	N=11	N=11

* 1 = Control groups; 2 = Experimental groups
** Analysis of variance, $p<.01$
*** Paired T-test, $p<.01$

staples they have learned about at the clinic. This is confirmed by the results in Table 22 for the protein index and the staple index. On both measures there are significant increases, both two units large. Since the possible range of the staple index is only half that of the protein index it can be said that the increase in choices for the first is comparatively larger.

The analysis up to now has not differentiated between mothers of different ethnic backgrounds. It is, however, quite likely that the cultural background of the mother is of considerable importance in the way in which she perceives the teaching and what she will accept of it.

The size of the groups does not allow for detailed breakdowns, and the following analysis will draw a comparison only between Ganda mothers and mothers from other tribes. This division splits the groups into subgroups of nearly equal size and is particularly warranted by the fact that the clinic is situated in the middle of Buganda, home of the Baganda, and that the other mothers must all be immigrants, either recent or of only one or two generations ago. The teaching, furthermore, is based largely on the foods familiar to the Baganda.

Ethnic background

This analysis will be confined to the protein and staple indices because they tell us basically all we want to know (Table 23). Among the outpatients, when first attending, the Ganda mothers score higher on both indices; but they show only small increases with education, and neither of these differences is significant. The outpatients from other tribes significantly increase their preferences for high-protein sauces to a level comparable to that of the Ganda control group. Like the Ganda mothers they show a minor shift in staple preferences. These results are far from heartening because the only significant change among the outpatients occurs in the preference for high-protein sauces among the tribes other than the Baganda, and they reach only the level of the Ganda women at their first attendance with a malnourished child.

As we already know from the previous discussion, the results with the inpatients are more positive in that the preference for high-protein sauces increases among both the Ganda and the other mothers.[19] In this case the increase in score of the Baganda is higher than that of the mothers from other tribes, a reversal of the finding among the outpatients. Both groups of mothers show large, comparable shifts in preferences towards plantain and sweet potato.

6.4 Conclusion

What are the differences between the teaching at the outpatient department and the teaching at the inpatient ward that may explain the previous findings? The first difference, of course, is that the IP course is much more intensive, that these mothers are more consistently exposed to the teaching. This may explain the greater magnitude of the changes achieved in the IP ward but not the qualitative differences. A second distinction between the two courses is that the inpatient mothers prepare the food for the children themselves. Handling the staple foods that are provided, they learn about them at least as much as, and perhaps more than, about high-protein sauces. This could explain why changes in staple preferences were found among the inpatients and not among the outpatients. One might, however, expect such a trend to occur more strongly among the mothers from other tribes since the Ganda mothers are already familiar with these staple foods, but this is not the case. There are other difficulties in interpreting the differences between Ganda and other women. Among the outpatients, Ganda mothers show no increase in preference for high-protein sauces, whereas the other mothers show significant changes in this respect. Among the inpatients, on the other hand, the Ganda mothers show a greater increase on this index than the mothers from other tribes. The question arises whether the distinction on the basis of tribe has been very relevant. Perhaps a distinction between urban and rural mothers would have been more illuminating. After all, it may well be that as regards the problems of child feeding, the difference between urban and rural conditions is more important than that between Baganda and other tribes. For this reason, we have concentrated on rural-urban differences in the analysis of the role of social factors as presented in Chapters 8 and 9.

What should be inferred from the finding that the inpatients show a strong shift in preference towards the staple foods that are used at the clinic? This is certainly not the intention of the teaching, but that does not necessarily mean that it should be judged negatively. There are, however, several disadvantages attached to such a shift. Firstly it is a change towards staple foods that contain less calories and less proteins (see Table 1, page 21). Also, and this applies probably most to mothers living in urban circumstances (who should be quite numerous among the women from the other tribes), it is a shift towards foods which are not only more difficult to prepare and store but which are often expensive and subject to seasonal shortages, in particular plantain. It certainly shows that the mothers learn little of the value of different staple foods and one wonders whether the policy of not saying anything detrimental about the traditional staple does not, in this instance, prove to be counterproductive. In all it is a shift that we do not feel happy about but it could perhaps be easily - and quietly - corrected by introducing other staple foods besides the two that were so much in use. In general it is probably better to pursue diversification rather than uniformity of foods, not only because it is nutritionally sound, but also because it will make the families less vulnerable in case of crop failure or other food shortages.

7 Teacher Training Colleges

The previous chapters have concentrated on nutrition education for women with young children. In the view of many writers, programmes such as these suffer the disadvantage that they tackle the problem after it has already come into existence: it would be better to teach people about feeding small children even before they have that responsibility. Teaching school children some of the basic elements of child nutrition is one example. Where a good proportion of all children attend school this seems sound, although few would deny that this approach has several, potentially severe, weaknesses (Scotney, 1976). The amount the children learn will be governed by the knowledge and motivation of their teachers, many of whom, especially at the primary school level, have themselves had a rather limited education. In the following study the knowledge and attitudes of this last group were assessed with the help of the methods used in Study 1.

The structure of education in Uganda was such that students entering teacher training colleges represent the middle range of primary school leavers; the best go on to secondary schools, the mid range typically enter teacher training colleges, while the remainder return home or take jobs. The group of recent entrants to teacher training colleges in all likelihood presents the medium level of nutritional knowledge and attitudes among primary school leavers. They also provide a base-line against which to compare the graduands after their four years' stay at these boarding colleges, before the large majority of them take up teaching posts in the primary schools throughout Uganda.

7.1 Study 3: method

The present study was conducted at four teacher training colleges within a fifty mile radius of Kampala. During the academic year 1971–2 the first-year students who had recently begun their training course and the fourth year students who were about to graduate were interviewed. Two colleges trained female, two trained male, teachers. This gave 104 male and 100 female first-year students, and 91 male and 112 female fourth-year students, or 407 in all. Few students leave the colleges before graduating, and Table 24 shows that both the total number of students and the composition of the two groups do not differ.

The students completed questionnaires in their classrooms, the questionnaire being closely modelled on the interview schedule used in the previous studies. Two of the scales, food knowledge and high-protein meals (see Appendix B) were identical to those used previously. The evaluative and dynamic ratings of matooke are also identical except that it was now possible to use 7-point, instead of 5-point, scales because of the paper and pencil format. On this occasion the sauce ratings (see Appendix B, page 132) were also included in the results, for reasons which will become clear later on. Two new knowledge scales were included. The first consisted of a list of four symptoms, two of which are characteristic of kwashiorkor (red hair, swollen legs), while the other two were not (heavy cough, yellow eyewhites). For each symptom the

Table 24. *Study 3. Composition of different groups of students at teacher training colleges*

	First year (N=204)	Fourth year (N=203)
Tribe: Ganda (percentage)	76	78
Median age (years)	16.0	20.7
Sex: male (percentage)	51	45

students had to indicate whether it was usually present in kwashiorkor patients, and scores could range from 0 to 4. The second new scale, immunization, simply asked the students to write down three diseases which could be prevented by immunization. Each correct answer counted for one point, so that scores on this scale could range from 0 to 3.

Table 25. *Study 3. Mean scores (and standard deviations) for students at teacher training colleges*

	First year (N=204)	Fourth year (N=203)
Symptoms of malnutrition	3.2 (0.9)	3.3 (0.7)
Food	2.8 (0.9)	2.7 (0.9)
Immunization	1.6 (1.0)	2.3* (0.8)
High-protein meals	4.7 (2.3)	5.1 (2.2)
Matooke: Evaluative	26.4 (6.3)	23.9** (7.5)
Dynamic	13.7 (5.7)	12.3 (5.8)
Sauce: Evaluative	30.4 (4.7)	28.7** (5.9)
Dynamic	17.5 (4.8)	16.1** (5.0)

* χ^2; $p < .001$

** Kolmogorov-Smirnov; $p < .05$

7.2 Results

As regards the three knowledge scales, symptoms, food and immunization, only the last shows a significant contrast between the first- and fourth-year students (Table 25). Clearly something was learned about immunization during the time at the colleges. The other knowledge scales, however, indicate virtually no difference between the groups. Comparing these students with the mothers in the first study (see Tables 7 and 12, on pages 66 and 71), it appears that the score of the students on the food knowledge scale (identical in the two studies) is similar to that of the regular attenders at Luteete and the inpatients at discharge from Mwanamugimu. As regards knowledge of malnutrition, a direct comparison between students and mothers is not possible because different questions were used, but it may be noted that on this topic scores averaged 80 per cent or more of the maximum score in both groups. To some extent it is reassuring that the knowledge of the primary school leavers surpasses that of the mothers who were presenting malnourished children at Mwanamugimu. During their four-year stay at the teacher training colleges, however, little or nothing is gained in this respect. This, certainly, is disappointing since one might have hoped that final-year trainee teachers would know considerably more than rural women with little formal education, especially as the students are more accustomed to tests and questionnaires.

A comparison of the two groups of students on the number of high-protein meals chosen indicated a slight, but statistically not significant, contrast between them, falling in the expected direction. This increase is smaller than that shown by the groups interviewed at the Mwanamugimu IP ward and at Luteete. The first-year students attain a score which is comparable to that of the control groups at these clinics and even falls below the score of the Mwanamugimu OP control group which consisted, after all, of mothers who had not succeeded in preventing malnutrition to occur in their children. Moreover, the mothers who had passed through these clinics gave more adequate responses than the fourth-year students.

The evaluative and dynamic ratings of matooke do show a difference between the two groups of students; both are lower in the group of graduands. This could be regarded as a hopeful sign, were it not that this change does not result from any increased nutritional insight. This, at least, is our interpretation of the finding that a similar decrease occurs in the two ratings of sauce. This general decrease in the ratings could possibly reflect a lower appreciation of the traditional foods, or else an increased ability to make refined judgements. Whatever the explanation of this finding, it cannot be regarded as a positive change in nutritional attitudes. Since the mothers used 5-point rating scales and the students 7-point scales, a direct comparison of the mean scores is not possible. When, however, the mean scores are expressed as a percentage of the maximum possible score, the results for the first-year students and the three control groups in the first study are remarkably similar. On the evaluative rating of matooke the first-year students score 73 per cent of the maximum score, the three control groups score 80 per cent, 68 per cent, and 71 per cent respectively. The same picture is presented by the dynamic rating of matooke: 57 per cent of the maximum score for the first-year students and 61 per cent, 58 per cent, and 56 per cent for the three groups of mothers. This confirms that these first-year students are not different in their nutritional attitudes from those rural women who had not been exposed to the teaching at the three clinics.[20]

7.3 Discussion

The comparison of the two groups of students has shown remarkably little contrast. The one exception is an increase in knowledge relating to immunization against diseases. Although it indicates an increase in health knowledge, this last finding cannot be considered a gain in nutritional knowledge. Such gains, apparently, do not occur at the teacher training colleges where there also are no signs of improved nutritional attitudes. In Chapter 1 we mentioned that it is left to the colleges to decide the extent to which they will cover nutrition, and that, if it is covered at all, the topic is scattered over different courses. This policy apparently leads to an absence of any increase in nutrition knowledge or improvement in attitudes, at least as reflected by these measurements.

When comparing the students with the women first attending the clinics in Study 1, the first-year students were found to have a better level of knowledge. Their scores on the attitude scales are, at best, similar to those obtained by these women. Nevertheless, their relatively good knowledge when leaving the primary schools indicates that some kind of basis was laid there, which makes it all the more regrettable that this is not followed up at the colleges. When leaving their colleges to take up places as primary school teachers, their nutritional knowledge does not surpass that of women who have received some nutrition education at the clinics and their attitudes are of a level comparable to that of rural women who have not been exposed to such nutrition education. It does not appear that these young primary school teachers will be able to contribute greatly to nutrition education among the children they will teach. In commenting on the situation in many developing countries Scotney has noted that 'Health education in the schools of less developed countries has frequently been very unsatisfactory. Programmes have been started and quietly dropped. Related subjects like hygiene and health sciences have been criticized as not being sound science and have not made headway . . .' (1976, p. 82.) Scotney continues by giving possible reasons for this failure, and among others, suggests that 'The schools aim at academic achievement and preparation for employment whereas health education is related to preparation for living and for citizenship . . . School systems have been built on European models. The good progress made in school health education in America and elsewhere has had little influence so far.' (1976, p. 82.) The results obtained in this study confirm that the teacher training colleges contribute little to a detailed understanding and appreciation of the local foods.

8 Environment and Recovery I

Previously it was demonstrated how between 25 and 30 per cent of the variations in nutritional status or recovery of the children attending the outpatient clinics could be attributed to variations in knowledge and attitudes of the mother of the child (see Chapter 5, page 73). The question arises as to what is responsible for the remaining variation. Part of it must be due to imprecision in the respective measurements; not only in the knowledge and attitude scales, but also in the weight measures which are often recorded under circumstances that are not conducive to making precise measurements.

Another source of variation lies in the actual behaviour of the mother which is decided only partly by her attitudes and knowledge, but also (perhaps to a larger extent) by different aspects of her environment. These may either support or restrict her in implementing what she has been told. The study of such extraneous influences is also part of 'process evaluation' and is the concern of the two following chapters. First we briefly review what is known about the social causes of malnutrition in Uganda. The two factors that are most often mentioned in the literature are poverty and instability of family relations[21] and, since outpatients convalesce at their homes, these same factors may presumably also be influential during recovery.

The role of poverty in causing malnutrition in Uganda is often considered as self-evident, but there are, in fact, few data to support this view. Welbourn (1955), in a study of 65 kwashiorkor patients, reported that none of the families of these children appeared poorer than its neighbours while many of the families were comparatively well-to-do. In another study, the poverty of the family was considered an important cause in only 4 out of 28 kwashiorkor patients (Farmer, 1960). The relation between socio-economic level and childhood malnutrition was studied in more detail among the Adhola in Bukedi district. Families that were well-to-do, according to their cash income, were found to have a greater consumption of high-protein relishes, a lower consumption of green vegetables, and fewer occasions on which no relish was served at all (Sharman, 1972). Despite this positive relationship between socio-economic level and protein consumption by the family, no association was found between socio-economic level and the nutritional status of the children. Malnourished children were just as frequent among the well-to-do families as they were among the poorer families. This lack of evidence for a relation between socio-economic level and childhood malnutrition is not surprising when it is realized that in a rural, subsistence economy, nearly every family grows its own food and that poverty eludes measurement. It may be argued that among immigrants, such as the Rwanda and the Luo, poverty is of a different nature because these groups have less access to land. They are less able or unable to grow their own foods, and since they are dependent on the cash economy they are, in fact, worse off than people who manage to grow their own foodcrops. Indeed, some studies point to a somewhat higher incidence of malnutrition among the Rwanda but not among the Luo (Brown and Opio, 1966; Welbourn, 1959).

Sending children to live with relatives at an early age is another factor often mentioned as a cause of childhood malnutrition, but it appears that two different practices have frequently been mistaken (Ainsworth, 1967, p. 418). Traditionally, among the Baganda, the child was sent to the grandmother at weaning, but returned to the mother after one or two nights to ensure its well-being. The other practice is to send the child away later in life to live with relatives for various (not necessarily negative) reasons. Evidence suggests that between 7 per cent and 22 per cent of kwashiorkor patients who were seen at a hospital, a dispensary, and a nutrition unit, were living away from their parents (Farmer, 1960; Brown and Opio, 1966; Schneideman *et al.*, 1971).

Welbourn (1959) observed that the practice was limited largely to Baganda children. She found that of 24 Baganda children who were severely malnourished, 11 (46 per cent) were living away from home, while this was the case for only 23 (9 per cent) of 248 Baganda children who attended child welfare clinics. (This last group contained relatively more children who were living in town.) In fact, in another study it was found that in a rural area a much larger proportion, i.e. 26 per cent, of the children were living with relatives (Welbourn, 1963). From these studies it is not clear whether the children were being sent away voluntarily or whether the separation coincided with a separation between the parents.

Marital instability is often mentioned as a contributing factor on its own. Where father and mother are separated or where a child is born out of wedlock, a cohesive family is presumably lacking, which will have negative consequences for the child. Although such reasoning tends to overlook the network of family relations and obligations upon which an individual in an African society can often rely, the suggestion warrants closer examination. Two studies reported an incidence of at least 14-19 per cent of broken marriages among the parents of kwashiorkor patients (Farmer, 1960; Brown and Opio, 1966). A much higher incidence of broken families, nearly 37 per cent, was found among the children attending the N.R.C. at Kampala (Schneideman *et al.*, 1971). It is not clear whether the different authors have used the same definition of a broken family, while comparable data for non-malnourished children are, unfortunately, lacking. In only one study was such a comparison drawn and it was found that the parents of 9 out of 65 kwashiorkor patients (14 per cent) had separated, but this was the case among only 35 out of 507 well-nourished children (7 per cent) (Welbourn, 1963).

Although the previous evidence is not conclusive, it appears that three social factors play a role in causing malnutrition. These are: (a) poverty, particularly among immigrants; (b) the practice of sending the child to live with relatives, in particular among the Baganda; and (c) marital instability. Whether they play a similar role during recovery remains to be seen, although this is usually the assumption. At Mwanamugimu information on the home and social background of the cases was routinely recorded to identify

Table 26. *Data recorded on the case files at Mwanamugimu N.R.C.*

Personal data on the mother:
- Name
- Address
- Distance to the Clinic

Date of admission
Date of birth of the child
Sex of the child
Data on the parents:
- Tribe
- Religion
- Alive or dead
- Marital status of the mother
- Marital situation: polygamous or monogamous

Data on the child and his siblings:
- Birth rank
- Does this child have a younger sibling?
- Has any other sibling had kwashiorkor?
- How many siblings have died?
- Is the mother pregnant?

Who is caring for the child?
Who brings him to the clinic?
How long ago did the mother stop breast feeding this child?
What other illnesses has the child suffered:
- Measles?
- Whooping cough?
- Ascaris?
- Hookworm?

What was the malnutrition diagnosis:
- Kwashiorkor or Marasmus?

What was the severity of this condition?

individual social problems. This information, summarized in Table 26, was collected in an interview with the mother as she first attended the clinic.

Robinson (1971) had previously studied these records but with little success. He selected 55 children who recovered well and compared them with 32 children who showed no catch-up growth but found that there was remarkably little difference between the two groups with respect to tribe, birth rank of the child, incidence of polygamous fathers, child not staying with his mother, unmarried mothers, and pregnancy of the mother. However, it does not necessarily follow from these results that the home environment of the child is not important in recovery. For one thing, the results of this study were marred by the fact that the data in the files related to the family situation of the mother, whether or not the child was actually staying with her. This means that for the children who were living away from the mother, the recorded information was largely irrelevant. But it is even more likely that the relationships are too complex to be revealed by the contrasting of extreme groups.

For these reasons, we decided to make a further attempt at studying these records, developing a more sensitive measure of recovery, including more children in the analysis, and also making more detailed comparisons.

8.1 Study 4: case records

The records of the 1171 outpatients who first attended during the year 1969 were abstracted in the spring of 1971, by which time at least one full year had elapsed since first attendance. In order to measure the child's progress adequately only those cases were selected who had attended at least four times over a period of two months (progress was quantified as in Study 1; see Appendix A). In all, 598 cases did not make four visits within the required period. In another 287 cases insufficient information on the child's age had been recorded, while for 8 cases the recorded weight data were incomplete, so that for these children also recovery rates could not be calculated. The files of another 7 cases were missing. Also left out were 69 cases living away from their mother, for whom no relevant information had been recorded. This left 202 cases out of the original total of 1171. Evidently this was a selected group, but the selection tended towards mothers who reattended regularly and who regarded the service given by the centre as relevant and helpful. Since attendance took time and money for transport, these must have been the women who felt that the centre had something to offer.

8.2 Rural vs. urban cases

In Chapter 6 a distinction was drawn between Ganda mothers and mothers from other tribes, but it was found that such an analysis gave little extra information. We therefore suggested that a distinction between 'rural' and 'urban' cases was perhaps more useful. Research on change processes in Africa has shown that the distinction between rural and urban living conditions is profound, and is related to other distinctions such as 'traditional' and 'modern'. Southall has described how the position and role of women alter radically with the move to Kampala, suggesting that this may represent a 'total and permanent break from rural and tribal society' (1961, p. 224.) For that reason, the 202 children were divided into a group of 87 children living in rural areas or in small villages, and a group of 115 children living in large towns (principally Kampala).

There are important differences in the tribal identity and the family circumstances of these two groups. In general the local Baganda live in the rural areas, whereas many immigrants, such as the Luo from Kenya, live in town. Marriage is virtually the rule among the Luo, with 96 per cent married; while for the rural Baganda the situation is more flexible, with only 80 per cent married. The mean family size in the rural areas is slightly larger, with an average number of 3.2 children compared with 2.8 in town. Finally there are more polygamous husbands in the rural group than in the town group. Data from the next study, presented in Chapter 9, confirm this. In general the extended families are to be found in the rural areas, while people in town tend to live in smaller family units.

The relation of these variables to recovery for both urban and

Table 27. *Study 4. Average recovery scores for urban cases compared with rural cases, by tribe and family (202 cases: those living with their mother)*

		Urban (N=115)		
Overall recovery		5.04		
Tribe of the mother	Ganda	4.07	others	5.18
Family	married	5.08	unmarried	4.75
	monogamous	5.16	polygamous	4.74
	1 or 2 children	5.05	3+ children	5.04
		Rural (N=87)		
Overall recovery		4.86		
Tribe of the mother	Ganda	4.92	others	4.79
Family	married	4.72	unmarried	5.75
	monogamous	4.76	polygamous	4.84
	1 or 2 children	4.41	3+children	5.15

rural groups are shown in Table 27. Town and country differ little in mean recovery scores, but within each group different variables appear to be associated with recovery. The Ganda children who live in town recover poorly. This may relate to the problems confronting the individual Ganda mothers, of whom in town only 50 per cent are married. Otherwise, the child may not be fed adequately because of the difficulty of cooking plantain and its high price in the urban areas, whereas other tribes often use other staple foods. In the rural areas the association between tribe and recovery is, if anything, reversed: the children of Ganda families recover slightly better than do the immigrant children.

The associations between recovery and selected aspects of family life also show intriguing patterns. In town, for example, it appears that the small, nuclear family gives a better prognosis than the larger, traditional family. The reverse appears to hold in the country, where children from large families (three children or more) recover considerably better than those from smaller families. It is possible that in the large, extended family the mother may find more help in caring for the child, and this may also be at the root of the curious finding that in the rural group children of unmarried mothers recover so much better than the children of mothers who are married and who should be able to rely on their husbands. Unmarried women in the rural areas will commonly stay with supporting relatives, forming a large family unit. The mother then becomes a relatively free agent; perhaps able to marshal considerable resources in the support of her child.

The overall impression gained from these results is that in terms of recovery from malnutrition, the 'modern', nuclear family has advantages in town, while the extended, 'traditional' family holds advantages in the country.

8.3 The relation between mother and child

One factor that has been stressed by many writers is that of the separation between mother and child (Jelliffe and Dean, 1959; Bennett, Lutwame and Namboze, 1963). The closeness of the African mother and her child during the first period of the child's life has been documented extensively. The first drastic separation from the mother usually occurs with weaning which among some tribes may be sudden and harsh. Depending upon the beliefs regarding pregnant women, the psychological 'distance' between mother and child may further increase when she becomes pregnant again. When the next sibling is born, this child takes the dominant position in the mother's attention.

Do these different stages of separation relate to recovery from malnutrition? Average recovery rates were computed for four groups of children: those at the breast, those weaned but whose mothers were not pregnant, those with pregnant mothers, and those with younger siblings. A distinction was once again drawn between Baganda and other tribes so as to be able to explain a drop in recovery scores among children whose mothers were pregnant, a finding which will be discussed later (Figure 4). In general, however, the greater the separation from the mother, the better the recovery of the child. These differences cannot be attributed to age differences between the groups because recovery

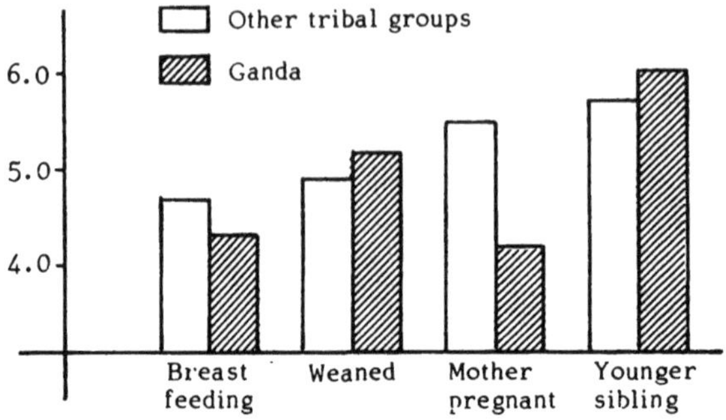

Figure 4 *Study 4. Average recovery score for different groups (N=202, children living with their mothers)*

rates were computed independent of age, but the following explanation is suggested.

A child that is still breastfed relies largely on its mother; if she is busy with other work or if her milk is failing, he is not able to find alternative sources of food. To the extent that the child becomes separated from his mother, he is also less dependent on her. Possibly the support from other family members, as well perhaps as the greater mobility of the child itself, result in faster recovery. A study by Albino and Thompson (1956) throws an interesting light on this. In South Africa, Zulu children are breastfed on demand until they are 18-24 months old, when on a certain day the mother smears her breast with the bitter juice of the aloe. After observing a group of children that were abruptly weaned in this way, the authors report that, quite naturally, the relationship between mother and child was initially unbalanced. What is interesting is that, contrary to expectations, these children showed no change in developmental level: rather, they soon displayed more independent behaviour and greater self-reliance, which was characterized by greater aggressiveness. In regard to feeding this may well imply that the child becomes more able to fend for himself.

Figure 4 shows that there is little difference between the Baganda and the other tribes except that, when the mother is pregnant, Ganda children recover considerably less well. The Baganda traditionally hold a strong belief in the harmful effects of a pregnancy for the youngest child, and they hold this to be a possible cause for what is called malnutrition. Many African peoples recognize a negative relation between the health of a child and the birth of the next one, but few are as explicit as the Baganda who hold that the 'heat' of the unborn child in the womb of the mother actually harms the elder sibling. Apparently, among the Baganda, the deleterious effects of a pregnancy also operate during recovery from malnutrition. Probably, and sadly, the pregnant Ganda mother may, for the sake of the child himself, tend not to pay much attention to him.

One common traditional solution to the problem of a pregnant mother caring for a young child was to send the child away to stay with a relative. This has commonly been discouraged by the nutrition education schemes because such a relative may not be highly motivated to care for someone else's child. And, indeed, as mentioned earlier in this chapter, there is reason to believe that this practice may contribute to the *occurrence* of malnutrition. But once they are living with relatives, it may be better to leave children (at least the Ganda children) there. In fact, the 69 children who were staying with relatives and who were not included in the above analysis recovered remarkably well. The mean recovery score for the 40 Ganda children in this group is high, at 5.52, while the mean score for the children from other tribes is also good, at 5.21. However, these children were among the most severely malnourished when first seen, which makes it possible for them to attain higher recovery rates than children with less serious weight deficits. Nevertheless, they must have been well cared for to enable them to sustain such good recovery scores. The assumption that leaving a child with relatives during his recovery has negative effects is not supported by these data.

The previous results indicate that the home environment of the child is certainly of importance during recovery from malnutrition, but that the factors which are often regarded as important in causation do not necessarily have that same influence during recovery, at least not among the regular attenders at the clinics.

9 Environment and Recovery II

In order to study the dynamics of recovery in more detail, one needs a framework or model that outlines which influences are important and how they apply. An initial step in building such a model, illustrated by Figure 5, is a series of hypotheses postulating how nutritional, economic, and social factors may influence the recovery of the child.

1. For a child to recover from protein-energy malnutrition and to sustain growth, he or she must consume adequate amounts of an appropriately balanced diet. Failure to recover may, however, also be due to illnesses, such as infections, but also including parasites or inadequate hydration. The rate of recovery is related to both these influences, and, by its nature, nutrition education concentrates mainly on the diet.

2. The adequacy of the diet for the malnourished child is determined by (a) the available food resources, which to a large extent are decided by the economic situation of the family; (b) the way these food resources are distributed among the members of the family; and (c) the suitability of the methods used for preparing the food and feeding it to the child.

3. The food resources are of three main types: (a) foods grown; (b) foods bought; and occasionally (c) gifts of food (for example, dried skimmed milk).

4. The way these resources are distributed among the family members and the suitability of the cooking and feeding methods that the mother uses will depend upon her knowledge and attitudes and upon the amount of time she has available.

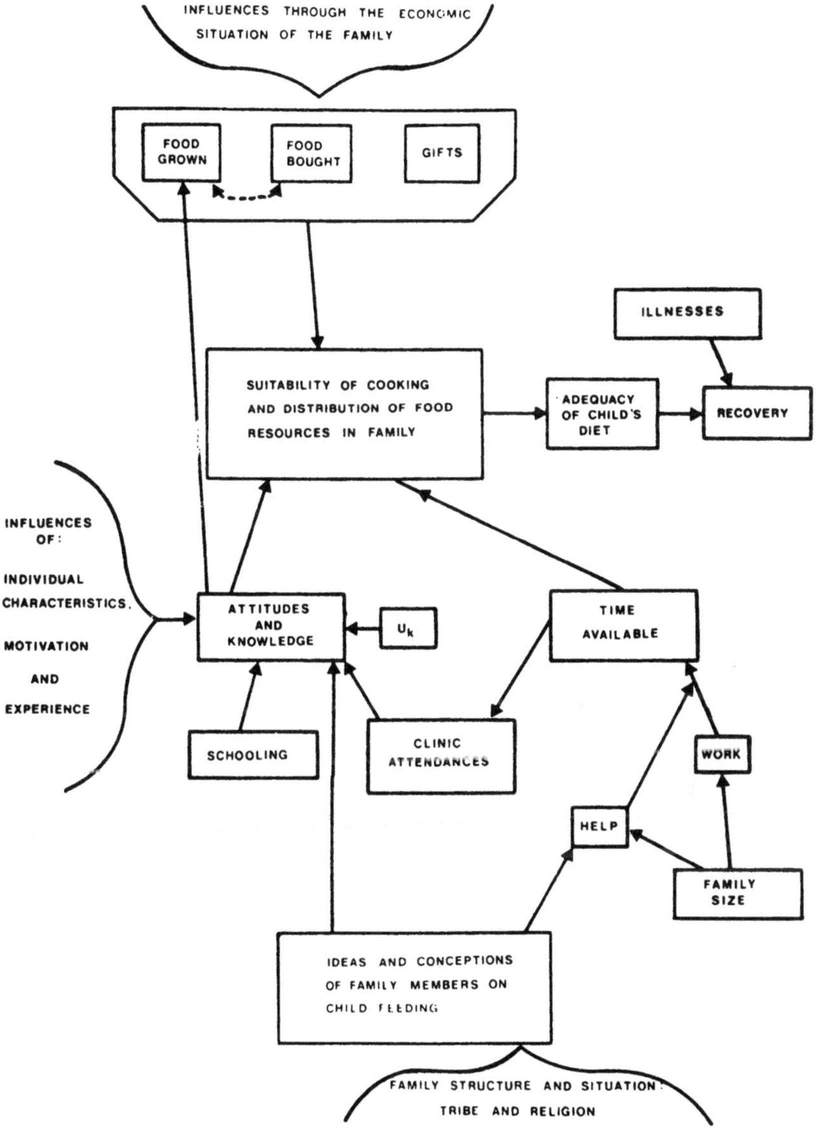

Figure 5. *The influence of the social environment on outpatient recovery from malnutrition*

5. Nutrition education concentrates on the mother's knowledge and attitudes which to some extent are also determined by any formal education she has received at school. These are by no means the only sources of information and a residual term (u_k) must be added. This part of the model reflects the individual mother's ability, experience, and motivation; but she is also influenced by the ideas and conceptions that her daily environment holds.

6. The amount of time the mother is able to spend on the cooking for, and the feeding of, the child varies according to how much work she has to do. If she has help in the household the possibility of catering separately for the child is increased as is the number of visits she can make to the clinic. Generally, in Africa a positive relation can be postulated between size of the family and the amount of help the mother receives.

The above can be illustrated concretely with the contrasting histories of three mothers who were attending Mwanamugimu outpatient clinic at the time.

The first mother lived 21 miles north of Kampala with her husband and only one child. They owned their own home and grew all the main vegetables, as well as staple foods and some cash crops. Although she was separated from a previous husband, the mother had lived with the father of this one child since it was born. She received help from a labourer on the farm and had the time to feed the child in the way taught at Mwanamugimu. The family did not have to pay any rent or school fees, and they could afford to buy meat, fish, and milk to supplement the foods grown on the farm. Since the child was recovering well the neighbours had taken an interest in what the mother had learned, and this encouraged her to continue in this way. Her husband provided money for transport to come to Mwanamugimu for follow-up appointments, and the mother herself seemed very content with the good progress of her child.

The second case provides an instance where the child was not recovering well, and many features of this case are the opposite to those of the first one. This mother had fallen on hard times. She had lived in her parents' home since leaving her husband, who had taken another wife; but clearly she had so much work to do that she could not adequately care for the child. The family owned $1\frac{1}{2}$ acres, all planted, and grew various vegetables. Since the recent death of the grandfather, there had been no wage earner in the family, and the grandmother was too old to help in the house or garden. The mother therefore had to care for her ageing mother, till the land, and look after the two children who lived with her. She herself was no longer young, having eight more children who were staying with various relatives. There was no one else nearby who could help her, although the neighbours were friendly and sympathetic. Nevertheless she seemed to try hard. She travelled quite far to attend Mwanamugimu as frequently as possible; and in order to supplement the children's diet she wove rush mats, but the income from this was irregular and meagre. The children were marginally nourished and suffered from frequent infections, the effect of which was exaggerated by their loss of appetite.

The contrast between the two cases is clear and relates to the regularity of the income, the stability of the home environment, and the existence of alternative food supplies. The time the mother is able to spend on the child is also important, as is the support or encouragement she receives. Another factor, however, is the personality of the mother and her determination to succeed. The women who lack such determination probably do not attend Mwanamugimu for long, if they attend at all.

Indeed, in certain cases the observer might well expect poor progress because of an indigent home environment, while in fact the mother manages to overcome her difficulties in remarkable ways. An example of such a case is the third mother who originally came from Rwanda but who now lived in a poor district in Kampala. Her husband had left home a year ago to look for a job. Since then she had experienced great problems in caring for her six children. Neverthelesss, she had succeeded remarkably; she bought tomatoes or charcoal cheaply, and sold these goods to her neighbours. Without any other means of support she was able to spend 25 shillings[22] per week on food as well as to pay 30 shillings rent per month. The child, as may be expected, was not recovering fast, but nevertheless was making some progress. It seems clear that with a less determined mother the child would have been doing less well. This last case also illustrates an important contrast between the families living in the town and those in the rural areas: the town dwellers are frequently immigrants, owning little or no land, and relying on a cash economy for their needs.

9.1 Study 5: design

Some of the ideas outlined at the beginning of this chapter and illustrated by the case histories were explored in a questionnaire study among a group of regular attenders at Mwanamugimu outpatient clinic. Each child's recovery was calculated in the same manner as in the previous case records study (see Appendix A) and therefore a minimum of 4 visits during the previous two months was required. It turned out that over the 10-week period of the study, starting from mid-march 1972, 64 cases in all were eligible. There were 31 boys and 33 girls in the group, and the mean number of previous visits was 9.8. Since they were to be subdivided into a 'rural' and 'urban' group as in the previous study, each group consisted of about 30 mothers and children.

In the case records study discussed in the previous chapter, the two subgroups had been distinguished solely by where they lived, whether in town or in the country. This was an attempt to distinguish the rural, agricultural, and traditionally African lifestyle from the town-dwelling, cash-economy, or modern situation. To reflect this contrast more closely, the cases in the present study were divided into two groups by considering four variables: distance to town, the amount of land owned, the type of family (nuclear or extended), and family size. Cross-tabulations indicated a close association between these four variables. By and large, cases fell into two groups: large, landowning families living some distance from the town; and small, or nuclear, families living near or in town. The only exception was a group of small, nuclear families who lived a considerable distance from town. As they were land-owners and probably represented young couples, they were included with the 'rural' cases. Although not adequate to cover the full extent of the contrast, the terms 'rural' and 'urban' will be used to describe these groups.

In the urban group 80 per cent of the women lived in nuclear families, while in the rural group 70 per cent were living in families with members of the third generation or other relatives present. The average number of children cared for by the mothers was 2.6 and 4.4 respectively. The groups also differed in an important associated characteristic. The local Baganda were predominant in the rural group, while immigrants (from Kenya, Rwanda, or other parts of Uganda) were found chiefly in the urban group. The mean recovery rate of the children was 5.5 for the rural cases and 5.0 for the urban cases. Although the rural children did slightly better, the rates for the two groups are comparable.

9.2 The questionnaire

Each woman participated for about 40 minutes in a semi-structured interview conducted in Luganda through an interpreter. In this interview many factors that are possibly influential in recovery were discussed, but particular attention was paid to the following seven aspects: the diet of the child, family resources, food resources, mother's experience and attitudes, household situation, support from others and tribe. The objection may be raised that several of these topics cannot satisfactorily be covered by questionnaire. We decided to rely on this method mainly because the first aim of the study was to develop a risk indicator which would also have to be taken by questionnaire (reported elsewhere; McDowell and Hoorweg, 1977). Part of the total information collected was coded into the 16 variables listed in Table 28 (see Section 9.3), each of the seven aspects being covered by up to three variables.

The adequacy of the child's *diet* is reflected by two variables: the first whether the recommended methods of food preparation were followed (var 1), the second whether the child generally had a good appetite or often refused food (var 2; the exact coding of the variables can be found in Note 23). The *resources* of most African families consist of the amount of land they have available and the cash income they derive from farming, jobs, etc. It is well nigh impossible to ask mothers at the clinic about land areas and incomes and to obtain reliable answers. Therefore we had to be satisfied with inquiring about the number of plots and whether they were permanently owned (var 3), which, of course, is only an approximation of the required information. Similarly we inquired after the number of sources of cash income (var 4). Assessing food resources posed similar difficulties. We therefore asked for the number of foods that were grown besides the staple foods (var 5), as these legumes and vegetables are usually kept for family consumption. An estimate of the amount of money usually spent on food during a week was also obtained (var 6). Lastly, because of its particular importance in child feeding and since it is often stressed in nutrition teaching, we inquired after the availability of milk (var 7), the more milk available the higher the score.

The *experience and attitudes of the mother* are reflected by her education (var 8) and the number of visits she has paid to the clinic (var 9). Furthermore, we applied an abbreviated paired-comparison scale that was somewhat different from the ones used previously. It resulted in a score, ranging from 0 to 9, of the high-protein meals preferred for a 2-year-old child (var 10). The *household situation* is reflected by the family situation (var 11) in which the scoring coped with a variety of situations, from a mother who had never been married and was living by herself through various alternatives to a woman who was permanently living with her husband. The size of the household (var 12) was also included, taking into consideration all the adults and children living in the home. The *support* the mother receives in caring for the child was ascertained by asking about the amount of help she received in her household duties (var 13), and also by inquiring whether her husband, if present (var 14), and her relatives (var 15) were informed about the teaching at the clinic and if so what were their reactions towards it. Finally the *tribe of the mother* was coded in such a way that the score increased with greater similarity to the general food habits of the Baganda to whom, after all, the teaching at the clinic is mainly geared.

Non-parametric correlations of each of these 16 variables with recovery were computed separately for the rural and the urban groups. For those variables that cover one particular aspect, multiple correlations were also computed, and these together with the single correlations are presented in Table 28.[24]

Table 28. *Study 5. Single and multiple correlations of different socio-economic variables with recovery*

	Rural (N=27)		Urban (N=37)	
1. Manner of food preparation	.14	.15	-.07	.09
2. Child's appetite	.11		.08	
#3. Land resources	.46*	.48	.08	.18
#4. Cash incomes	.20		-.13	
5. Foods grown	.16	.34	.11	.20
6. Foods bought	.30		.03	
7. Milk availability	.18		.14	
#8. Education of mother	.12	.17	-.49.	.54
9. Visits to clinic	.12		.05	
10. Attitude score	.14		.11	
11. Family situation	.08	.51	.27	.40
12. Size of household	.47*		.28	
#13. Household help	.45*	.47	.10	.48
14. Attitude of husband towards teaching	.12		.29	
#15. Attitude of relatives towards teaching	.13		.43*	
#16. Tribe	.10		-.48*	

* $p < .05$

Significant differences between the correlations in the urban and the rural groups; $p < .05$

9.3 Results and discussion

Among the rural group all correlations, whether small or large, are in the expected (positive) direction. This is not the case among the urban group, and it seems that in general terms the model as outlined at the start of this chapter is more relevant for the rural than for the urban situation.

In the rural group recovery shows significant correlations with the amount of land available to the family, the size of the household, and the help the mother receives. This closely confirms the findings of the previous study where it was also found that in the rural situation the large extended family gave the best chance for recovery.

Among the urban group the variable most strongly associated with recovery is the formal education of the mother. This association curiously is an inverse one: increased length of schooling is associated with poorer progress. Nearly equally important appears to be the tribal background, but the negative correlation indicates that in town Ganda children recover less well. Thirdly, a helpful attitude of the relatives (and of the father) also influences recovery.

In relation to the negative correlation of formal education with recovery among the urban women it must be noted that the 'higher' educated women in this group still had only 4 to 5 years of primary education. Perhaps they had developed certain attitudes without gaining the skills or means to fulfill them. The finding at least points to a conflict between school experience and what they are taught at the clinic. It may be that they regard the teaching as suitable for uneducated, rural women but not applicable to themselves since they have other ways of life, and possibly, other aspirations. (Perhaps these women are the ones most likely to spend their scarce resources on expensive Western types of food for their children.) These, then, are the high correlations that are observed.

Several variables, however, show low correlations with recovery in both the urban and rural group. These are, first, the two variables concerned with the diet of the child. To our view this lack of relationship must be attributed to shortcomings of the questions that were asked. It is also possible that many women may have tended to reply affirmatively irrespective of their real practices. (In general it is difficult to obtain reliable information on food preparation and consumption through questionnaires although a promising method has been described by Blankhart (1971).)

The three indicators of food resources also show low correlations with recovery and, again, we are inclined to attribute these low correlations not so much to an actual absence of relations as to the shortcomings of these questions which probably failed to assess the actual food resources. That the number of visits to the clinic *per se* bears no relation with recovery need not necessarily surprise us. On the one hand it may be expected that with more visits the women will learn more and implement more of that what is learned. On the other hand it is not unlikely that the mothers of cases that recover well will stop attending after a while but that the mothers of children that recover poorly will keep seeking help and advice. That the attitude score does not correlate with recovery indicates that the paired-comparison scale used was less adequate than that employed in the previous studies.

Apart from the actual magnitude of the correlations between individual variables and recovery, the differences between correlations in the urban and rural group are equally interesting because they show that different processes are at work in the two groups. The variables that show significantly different correlations can be found in Table 28 and are each discussed below.

Land resources are significantly correlated with recovery among the rural group, possibly more directly reflecting the food resources that are available to the family. In town, however, no such relation is present probably because townspeople in general have little access to land, so that there are few differences between them in the first place. In the second place, even when they own pieces of land outside the town, the proceeds of these are not available to them on a day-to-day basis so that the daily diet of the child can benefit but little from it.

As regards cash incomes, a positive relation with recovery, if it exists, exists more in the rural than the urban environment. Why that is, we can only speculate. Perhaps the level of income is so low, particularly in town, that it is insufficient to meet the primary needs of the family anyway, so that there is no surplus which can be used to buy foods for the sick child. Those people who actually buy foods for the child are not necessarily better off than others who do not, but may do so for their individual reasons. In the rural areas, however, incomes often are over and above the subsistence level and are apparently more predictive of recovery.

The inverse relation between formal education of the mother and recovery of the child does not hold for the rural women. Probably the rural educated women see themselves as rural women first and accept the teaching as relevant to their situation. Their reference group is that of the rural mothers, whether educated or not, and thus neither a negative nor a positive relation with education exists.

Household size and household help are both significantly correlated with recovery in the rural environment. The larger the family and the more help, the better the recovery; both of these relations do not hold in the urban environment. In the previous case records study we found that in town the nuclear type of family was more conducive to good progress than large extended families. This is not quite confirmed in the present study since we do not find a negative correlation with the *size* of the family among the urban group. However, there is a small positive association between recovery scores and living in a nuclear family among the urban cases.

Regarding support from others, the attitudes of the relatives and the father are clearly more important in town than in the country. This may again suggest the greater dependence of the woman on the husband in the urban, nuclear family situation. Since she is usually dependent upon her husband's income, his attitude and co-operation are probably very important. Why, however, the attitude of the relatives to the teaching is that much more important in town than in the country, we fail to understand, unless it is that in town the mother usually has such limited possibility of manoeuvering that she needs the active support of family members. Unless the mother receives such support, perhaps as part of a system of general adaptation to poverty, she may well be unable to cope successfully with the additional stress of caring for a sick child.

Finally, the finding that in town the children of the Baganda and tribes similar in food culture recover much less well - and that this is not the case among the rural women - confirms the same finding in the previous case records study.

9.4 Conclusions

To summarize, we may have a look at the multiple correlations between recovery and the subgroups of variables that assess each of the seven aspects on which this study concentrated. In the rural situation differences in family resources, household situation, and household help are important in determining the recovery of the malnourished child. In town the household situation and the help and the support from others are also important together with the educational level of the mother and her tribal background, findings which we have commented upon.

The present study is but an imperfect test of the model that was outlined at the beginning of this chapter because the number of subjects was rather small and because the questionnaire method that was employed has obvious weaknesses. Nevertheless, the results lend support to some of the hypotheses while also demonstrating that different processes are at work among the urban and rural mothers, processes that apparently are quite influential in the recovery of the child.

The implications for the operation of the nutrition centre are that teaching should be tailored more specifically to the situation in which the child is to be treated. The basic distinction should be recognized between rural and urban cases, that is the difference between large, extended families living on the land and small, nuclear families living in town. At the time of the study the same teaching was given to both groups. It stressed, for example, the need to grow certain crops, irrespective of whether or not the mother had access to land. Nutrition education for the urban mothers would appear to present a more difficult task than for the rural cases, because in town the important factor is probably poverty for which the clinic can do little. Mandeville (1974, p. 70) says of the urban Baganda that 'many people are completely dependent on money for all their wants, a fact which new arrivals evidently have some difficulty in fully grasping.' The major role of the nutrition rehabilitation centre, beyond teaching about suitable foods for the child, should lie in encouraging the mother to make the most of her resources. The important role that husband and relatives apparently play in the urban circumstances raises the question of whether more efforts should be made to reach them as well, rather than to concentrate on mother and child exclusively. Perhaps these husbands should be more actively encouraged to attend the clinic, or more emphasis should be placed on home visits by the staff, while the mother could also be recommended to seek the help of those relatives whom she has nearby.

10 Conclusions

It is now estimated that in many developing countries up to 5 per cent or 10 per cent of young children may suffer from severe protein-energy malnutrition at any one time, and that as many as 20 or 30 per cent, sometimes even 40 per cent, of the children suffer from moderate malnutrition (Bengoa, 1973; deMayer, 1976). Although this has given rise to great concern and has resulted in extensive research, not to mention numerous conferences, little actual progress has been made towards preventing the condition. 'The complexity of the problem has discouraged many health authorities from undertaking measures to alleviate its gravity; this is in contrast to the great progress that has been made in the prevention and treatment of so many other health problems' (de Mayer, 1976, p. 24.) Indeed, many argue that only improvements in the general level of living will significantly affect the incidence of malnutrition, and that priority should therefore be given to economic measures. However, as Berg (1973) has pointed out, malnutrition not only results from underdevelopment but also serves as one of its causes. Standards of living in most developing countries are not improving at a substantial rate, and even those countries which in previous years had satisfactory rates of economic growth did not show corresponding improvements in nutrition (Bengoa, 1973). Clearly, childhood malnutrition causes so much suffering that we cannot wait until it is alleviated by the process of economic development. Equally clearly, malnutrition will not be overcome without improvements in general standards of living, so that among the different kinds of intervention, nutrition education appears a logical approach. Teaching women how best to apply their resources may contribute to improvements in nutritional levels and, in some small measure, to economic and social development. It is exactly in this field that relatively little progress has been made. Although the efforts of individual health personnel are often exemplary, and although nutrition rehabilitation centres are an improvement over hospital care, these efforts remain severely hampered by a lack of information about how such teaching is received and what changes it brings about. As one author in a recent W.H.O. monograph, *Nutrition in Preventive Medicine,* emphasizes: 'At the present time the greatest void in nutrition research programmes is in the area of education: in teaching methods, both formal and informal and in methods for evaluating the results of educational efforts.' (Bosley, 1976, p. 294.) Demands for evaluative studies are widely expressed (Berg, 1973; Bain, 1973; Bengoa and Beaton, 1976; F.A.O./W.H.O., 1976), but there is a notable lack of suitable methods and of experience in this field.

10.1 Evaluative research

Nutrition education influences the nutritional status of a child not directly, but only through the intermediary of the mother. Education seeks to change her knowledge and attitudes and hence her behaviour, which may ultimately result in improved child health. Personal and social factors also influence a mother's attitudes, while her behaviour moreover depends on various social, economic, and (especially) family circumstances. The child's nutritional status in its turn is not only dependent upon feeding but is also closely related to the incidence of infections.

At present, most evaluation concentrates on assessing final results and is limited to measuring improvements in child health. Evaluative studies rarely investigate *why* the observed effects occurred, so that, apart from the measure of eventual success, little understanding is achieved. A more thorough type of evaluation, however, studies aspects of the entire process from the initial input, the education, to the final outcome, taking measures at each of the interjacent levels. As well as monitoring the child's health, this 'process' evaluation covers the knowledge, attitudes, and behaviour of the mother not only in relation to the education but also in combination with other social and economic variables. In that way insights can be gained from which improvements in education may emanate. The fact that such process evaluation is presently lacking in most nutrition programmes in developing countries inhibits the development of effective preventive measures, because of our inadequate understanding of the influences operating on the mother.

If the nutrition education of mothers of young children in developing countries is expected to contribute substantially to the prevention of malnutrition, it merits serious research beyond the evaluative shortcuts that are presently used. Admittedly such process evaluation faces great problems arising from the fact that programmes are often in full operation and that subjects and conditions can not be manipulated at will. This situation is not much improved by the occasional consultation of methodologists and social scientists who often strongly favour true experimental studies, usually a patent impossibility. It is to this stalemate that the present monograph addresses itself, exploring and demonstrating possible methods of investigation.

The studies reported here concentrate principally on the nutrition rehabilitation centre in Kampala. N.R.C.s increasingly take a central position in the provision of nutrition education in many developing countries. They are concerned mainly with malnourished children and their mothers, although in this they represent only one of a possible range of educational approaches. However, they meet malnutrition in its most severe forms and in that sense often serve as a cradle of experience.

The first aim of the present monograph is to form a contribution to methods of evaluative research. For this reason, rather than presenting any large-scale evaluation, it consists of a series of smaller studies into different aspects of the process by which education may help to treat and prevent childhood malnutrition. In the course of these studies, however, certain findings were reported that should be of interest to the more practically minded.

At the start of any evaluation two aspects of method have to be considered: first the question of the measurements or criteria that will be used, and secondly that of the research designs that are to be employed. We have argued that because of the conditions prevailing in most nutrition programmes in developing countries, there is a growing need for adequate, that is methodologically acceptable, and yet, at the same time, practicable designs. Quasi-experimental designs give far greater possibilities in this regard than the standard 'pretest-posttest' design, although their interpretation is often less straightforward and requires greater caution.

By assessing knowledge, and particularly by applying attitude measures, the researcher lays himself open to the criticism that it is not one of the aims of the education to influence mothers in this particular way, i.e. to gain improvements on a certain attitude scale. This situation will frequently be met by any researcher who does not evaluate strictly according to the 'stated objectives' but it is our conviction that in this lies exactly the contribution that social scientists can make. Whether the measurements themselves are adequate may to some extent be judged by first impressions; they are judged more accurately by other methods of reliability and validity assessment, and they are judged ultimately by the insights that are gained through their use.

The first studies reported in Chapters 4 and 5 of this monograph demonstrate how knowledge and attitude scales applied in 'posttest-only' designs were used in three nutrition programmes in Uganda. These three programmes are at the inpatient ward at the N.R.C. in Kampala, the outpatient department at the same centre, and a young child clinic at Luteete, a village some 40 miles from Kampala. The findings corresponded with the differences existing between the programmes. The rural clinic serves all young children. It pays considerable attention to child nutrition, but without placing as much emphasis on malnutrition as is done at the N.R.C.

The main content of the findings is discussed below. For small groups of outpatients it is demonstrated that the knowledge and attitude measures explain a sizeable part of the variation occurring in the recovery and nutritional status of these children. Having demonstrated the feasibility of these methods of evaluation, some findings are further explored. This second study shows that, apart from the expected changes in food choices, certain unintended learning processes occur among the mothers admitted to the IP ward which, in our opinion, need correction. This last study, in particular, provides an example of the detailed investigations that can be carried out in this way; such insights could never be gained from relying exclusively on weight data.

The premise of nutrition education is that mothers are, to some extent, lacking in knowledge, that their attitudes and practices are inappropriate, and that improvements in this respect will lead to improved child health. To what extent, however, do economic, social, and family circumstances impose restrictions and determine the improvements that are possible? In Chapters 8 and 9 two studies are reported that concentrate on the role of social and economic factors in the recovery of malnourished children. The first (Study 4) is based on the case records kept at the outpatient department of the N.R.C., the next (Study 5) based on interviews with mothers regularly attending the same clinic. The findings indicate that certain factors (notably mother-child separation and incomplete families) which are possible contributory factors to malnutrition, do not always exert a negative influence during recovery. It is usually assumed that the role of causative factors remains unaltered in the course of the disease and the following treatment. Both studies furthermore point to important differences in the social processes that promote good recovery among different groups of patients, classified as 'rural' and 'urban', although the average recovery rate of these groups is not noticeably different. This finding has serious implications for the operation of the centres, as discussed below, and emphasizes the need to include such studies as a part of process evaluation.

The present monograph forms an exploration in evaluative research, but the possibilities and the needs for further research are clear. First of all, there are other types of nutrition education that merit study. More important than the question of how different programmes compare is the question of how different programmes function in different ecological environments and how successful are different approaches with mothers living under different social and economic circumstances.[25] Behind these questions looms ultimately the question of selective intervention: how to aim different types of nutrition education, or more generally, different types of nutrition intervention, at those parts of the population to whom they are most suited and who will benefit most from them.

10.2 Findings and recommendations

A selection of the findings concerning the young-child clinic at Luteete and the nutrition rehabilitation centre at Kampala which were reported in Chapters 5, 6, 8, and 9 are briefly presented together with some recommendations.

The teaching at the three programmes has a positive effect on the knowledge of the mothers. The inpatients at the N.R.C. increase their knowledge about the disease of malnutrition and about the nutritional value of foods; the outpatients improve only their knowledge about the disease. At the rural young-child clinic, mothers increase their understanding of the nutritional value of foods but do not gain knowledge about the disease, partly because this is already quite high.

The teaching also leads to positive changes in patterns of preferences for meals for young children, with a growing tendency to select meals with a high protein content. In the first study the rural centre was the only programme where these changes were found to be statistically significant; among the inpatients at the N.R.C. they were substantial but not significant, while among the outpatients they were negligible.

The regular attenders at the rural centre score better on nearly all counts than the mothers who have attended the N.R.C. These high scores can be attributed only partially to a higher level of scores when these mothers first attend the rural clinic. Only in their level of understanding of the disease do they fall below the two groups at the N.R.C., but they know more about the nutritional value of foods than the N.R.C. outpatients and are equal to the N.R.C. inpatients in this respect. They perform, however, by far the best on the attitude measures, showing a greater preference for meals with a high protein content and rating steamed plantain lower both as regards its 'evaluative' and its 'dynamic' characteristics.

On the basis of these findings it appears that the rural young-child clinic is ultimately the most successful of the three programmes. This greater success is in part due to the fact that simply because the rural clinic is situated closer to the homes of the attendants, the mothers are able to attend more often and for longer periods of time than can the visitors to the N.R.C. Nutrition education has greater effects if given at the local level than when carried out at centralized clinics where those attending usually form a very mixed group of people. Those attending small rural clinics form relatively homogeneous populations, and they tend to know one another which probably makes them more at ease. At small rural centres the teaching can also more easily be adapted to the local circumstances. Another important factor at Luteete is the presence of an active social worker who visits most of the homes in the area. This creates ties with the families, ties that are very much harder to maintain from the central N.R.C., and which are absent from many other nutrition programmes. Whichever factor is most instrumental is difficult to say, although all probably contribute to the measure of success of this programme.

Further investigations at the N.R.C. reveal that both inpatients and outpatients show certain changes in their preferences for meals for small children. These changes towards foods with a relatively high protein content are significant in both groups but, again, are greater among the inpatients than among the outpatients. This difference between inpatients and outpatients in all probability results from the intensive experience provided by an inpatient course whereby the mothers not only undergo more teaching and receive more individual attention, but are also involved in the daily preparation of the meals.

The inpatients, furthermore, show an even greater increase in preferences for the two staple foods that are mainly used at the centre, plantain and sweet potato. This trend is largely absent among the outpatients, and therefore probably results from the fact that the inpatient mothers prepare their own meals and thus learn as much, if not more, about staple foods as they do about sauces. Since this is a shift away from more nutritious foods and probably further restricts the variety of staple foods that is used, we deem this trend unfortunate. It could be relatively easily corrected by relying less on these two foods and including other staple foods more often in both the teaching and the daily preparation of meals.

Although one possible cause of malnutrition lies with the practice, not uncommon among the Baganda, of sending children to live with relatives, there are no indications that chances for *recovery* are poorer for these children. This suggests that the policy of insisting that children must return to their mothers, if at all possible, should not be pursued in its present form. In particular, the poor recovery shown by Ganda children whose mothers are pregnant confirms the need for a reconsideration of this strategy.

Studies into the relation between recovery and social environment indicate that a fundamental difference should be made in treating the contrasting cases, whom we have characterized as 'rural' and 'urban'. In town the best prognosis for recovery appears to lie with those children who live in small, stable families. In the country the opposite is the case, and those children recover best who live in large families and in families who own sufficient land, while in these circumstances it is not important whether the mother is safely married or not. The teaching at the clinic is geared basically to the living circumstances and food practices of the rural Baganda and, for example, stresses the need to grow a variety of foods at the home. Such advice is of little use to a town-dwelling family with no land, although much of the other teaching remains useful. Nevertheless, the distinction between these groups should be recognized, and attention should be given to those groups known to show poor progress. In town these include first, the Baganda and related tribes such as the Banyankole, Banyoro, and Basoga; further, the relatively educated mothers, the large families, and the mothers who receive little support from their relatives and husbands. In the country poor progress is shown in small families, families who have little land available, and where the mother has no help in the household. A special group, of course, are the pregnant Ganda mothers already mentioned. It would be surprising if in combination these adverse conditions do not further decrease the chances for recovery of the child. Apparently the standard educational approach is not successful with these groups and alternatives must be considered.

First, and above all, it is important that these cases are recognized by the staff and asked to attend more often in order to be closely supervised. In the case of the pregnant Ganda mothers, individual counselling might help to counter the belief about the danger of close contact with the elder child. Individual counselling, however, offers no solution for the rural mothers with small families, with no help in the household, or with little land available. These are probably women with a heavy work load who are simply not able to get through the extra tasks which the recommended practices entail. Even asking them to pay more visits may be too much of a burden for them. It would appear that these cases could benefit greatly from admission to the inpatient ward where the mother can spend most of her time caring for her child. The urban cases that show poor progress could similarly benefit from admission to the inpatient department. For these last cases, however, the possibility might be considered of providing day care, whereby the mothers participate in the daily activities of the inpatients but spend nights at their homes. From several countries satisfactory results have been reported with this type of rehabilitation (Bengoa, 1976).

More attention should also be given in the teaching to the problems that face mothers in town. For example, in such cases the teaching might concentrate on the cheapest foods, on economical ways of cooking, on using left-overs, and so forth. In short, the aim of the teaching should more specifically be to help the mother adapt to urban living conditions without necessarily clinging to traditional food practices. This fits in with the previous recommendation about the use of more than two staple foods at the centre. Of course, such education for urban mothers is a difficult task, because one underlying factor is often poverty. One might consider whether in such cases the nutrition education should not be combined with the provision of supplementary foods. Preferably, such supplementation should not be limited to dried skimmed milk but should consist of a wider variety of foods. If this recommendation is ever taken up, we also suggest that the supplementation should not cease immediately after the recovery of the child, but continue for a period of several months.

This last section dealt with selective intervention among the attenders to this particular rehabilitation centre. It is our conviction that the most important contribution of evaluative research will be to enable the development of strategies for selective nutrition intervention.

APPENDIX A

Measuring Recovery Rate

The recovery rate of a malnourished child can be measured in several ways. Biochemical indices give an assessment of metabolic balance which is probably most useful in the assessment of the 'acute' condition (Hay *et al.,* 1975). Since the stunting of growth is a prominent feature of chronic undernutrition, height gain can potentially also serve as an indicator of recovery. Height increases very slowly, however, and in that sense it does not represent a sensitive indicator. (It must also be measured with great accuracy, and for that reason also is probably less suited to the conditions at most clinics.) It is therefore not surprising that weights are most commonly used as indicators of recovery. 'Outcome' studies of N.R.C.s usually assess weights in some way, but often classify the cases into only a few categories. This may be adequate, if and when enough cases are included. Yet when, as in the present studies, further statistical analysis is required, it becomes necessary to calculate individual recovery rates more precisely. However, just as height is a somewhat insensitive means to measure recovery over shorter periods, weight perhaps fluctuates too easily. Bodyweight depends, to a certain extent, on erratic influences such as whether the child has just eaten a large meal or not and is also rapidly influenced by bouts of infectious disease. For weights to be used as valid indicators of recovery, such fluctuations should be excluded. But even when they have been eliminated there are still several formulas that can be used to quantify the rate of growth, three of which will be discussed in more detail.

A.1 Three formulas

Formula 1. Grams per day

The first formula is the simplest and expresses the child's weight gains as a rate of grams gained per day:

$$\frac{\text{Weight gained during convalescence (grams)}}{\text{Duration of convalescence (days)}} \qquad (1)$$

A limitation to this formula is that it does not accommodate any of the various factors which may influence recovery rate differently at different ages. The normal growth rate of children varies with age; and the amount of food eaten by children of different ages varies, so that they may recover at different rates. There is some indication that children of different ages do recover at different rates. Garrow and Pike (1967) reported a positive relationship between the child's age and a clinical assessment of recovery velocity. Graham *et al.* (1969) note an increase in the rate of gain of cell mass during recovery with increasing age. Our own data, taken from outpatients at the N.R.C. at Kampala, also suggest a slight positive association between the age of the child and his recovery rate as measured by Formula 1. These findings make it desirable to control for the age of the child in calculating his recovery rate, where it is intended to compare the progress of children of various ages. Formula 1 does not allow for this.

Formula 2. Grams per kilogram bodyweight per day

An alternative formula exists which may control for the age of the child although it was not specifically designed for this purpose. In this case the weight gains are expressed as a proportion of the bodyweight of the child so that the weight gain of an older child is generally divided by a higher figure than that of a younger child:

$$\begin{matrix}\text{Weight gained}\\ \text{during convalescence}\\ \text{(grams)}\end{matrix} \Bigg/ \begin{matrix}\text{Bodyweight}\\ \text{(kg)}\end{matrix} \Bigg/ \begin{matrix}\text{Duration of}\\ \text{convalescence}\\ \text{(days)}\end{matrix} \qquad (2)$$

The rationale for this is that the older, heavier child can eat more, and his catch-up weight gains can be expected to be higher. This formula has been used by Ashworth, Bell, James, and Waterlow (1968); Ashworth (1969); and by Krieger and Chen (1969).

Formula 3. Comparison with the normal growth rate

An alternative modification to Formula 1 has been proposed, which aims at compensating for the different normal growth rates of children of different ages. It compares the recovery rate of each child with the normal growth velocity of children of that age, both rates (normal and recovery) being expressed in grams per day. The result may be calculated as a percentage, so that if the child is recovering his deficit, the score is more than 100 per cent:

$$\frac{\text{Weight gained/Time (for convalescing child)} \quad \text{(grams per day)}}{\text{Weight gained/Time (for normal child of same age)} \quad \text{(grams per day)}} \times 100 \quad (3)$$

This approach has been used by Prader, Tanner, and von Harnack (1963); Robinson (1971); and Schneideman *et al.* (1971). Church and Stanfield (1971) and King *et al.* (1972) use this method as the basis for a simple field measure.

Formula 2 and Formula 3 cannot be considered to be equivalent because they correct the absolute weight gains by different factors. That used in Formula 2 is the child's weight, while Formula 3 uses the normal growth rate. These correction factors are themselves negatively related. A young child will be low in weight, but has a high growth rate, while the opposite holds for an older child. Hence young children will tend to score high on Formula 2, while older children will tend to score high on Formula 3. This has in effect been demonstrated elsewhere (McDowell and Clayden, 1974) where it was shown that recovery rates for the same children computed with both Formula 2 and

Table 29. *Mean recovery values for young children compared with older children by formulae 2 and 3*

	Young children (8 to 18 months) (N=141)	Older children (>26 months) (N=95)	Significance level (t-test: two-tailed)
Formula 2: (Grams per kg. per day)	2.23	1.91	$p < .05$
Formula 3: (% of normal growth rate)	221.0	363.9	$p < .003$

Formula 3 give significantly different results for younger and older children (Table 29). Which formula gives the 'truer' result is hard to answer; certainly both are correlated with the age of the child, albeit in opposite directions. Neither gives a measure by which both younger and older children have an equal chance of attaining a high (or low) score. Therefore a new scoring system has been developed.

A.2 Standard recovery score

Recovery 'standards' for different age groups were calculated on the basis of the weight gains of 360 outpatients at Mwanamugimu. These constituted all the outpatients attending during 1969 and three months of 1972 who made at least four visits to the unit over a period of two months, and whose ages were known accurately. The children were of both sexes, and were aged between 7 and 70 months. They were divided into five age groups: below 12 months; 13-18 months; 19-24 months; 25-36 months; 37 months and over. These age ranges were chosen because within each of them the normal growth rate is almost linear, so that direct comparisons may be made between recovery rates within each group. Weights taken at visits when the child was reported to be suffering from infection (recorded by the medical assistant) were excluded. Next, a regression line was drawn through the steepest part of the remainder of each child's recovery slope, provided that this lasted for at least three weeks, so that the slope of the regression line expressed grams weight gained per day. (The steepest section was used on the principle that this represented the best rate of growth, free from illness, that the environment could sustain.)

Within each of the age groups these weight gains were ordered from the lowest to the highest. Next, the lowest 4 per cent of weight gains were allocated score 1; the lowest 5-11 per cent, score 2; etc.; as follows:

Score	*Percentage of cases*
1	lowest 4
2	5 to 11
3	12 to 23
4	24 to 40
5	41 to 60
6	61 to 77
7	78 to 89
8	90 to 96
9	highest 4

This produced a table of weight gains for each age group. With the help of these tables, weight gains in grams per day can be converted into standard scores ranging from 1-9. This scoring system is independent of age, since, for example, in each age group the 4 per cent of the children with the lowest recovery rates all score 1. It has the further advantage that extreme weight gains by certain children no longer exert an unduly large influence in computations. This recovery score was used throughout this monograph and is referred to as the 'recovery' score.

APPENDIX B

Measuring knowledge and attitudes

B.1 Knowledge questionnaire

A knowledge questionnaire should consist of factual questions which reflect, more or less closely, the actual content of the teaching. As described in Chapter 2 the teaching at the clinics, particularly at Mwanamugimu, concentrates on the recognition and causes of malnutrition, certain child-rearing practices, and the value of foods. Four groups of knowledge questions were finally drawn up (Table 6, page 61), after easier questions had failed to differentiate between respondents, because nearly everyone knew the correct answers.

Disease knowledge
The first group of questions concerns itself with the recognition and causes of both 'acute' malnutrition and 'chronic' undernutrition. The majority of a group of 97 mothers first attending the clinics (the groups labelled '1' in Table 4, page 58) replied correctly, particularly on the recognition questions, and slightly less on the causation questions (Table 30). The four questions together form a relatively stable scale, with coefficients of reproducibility and scalability of .84 and .52 respectively.

Child rearing knowledge
The three questions concerned with child rearing are all derived directly from the teaching. It is generally recommended to start additional feeding around the age of 5 months, to wean a child at

Table 30. *Knowledge questions (results for a group of 97 women first attending at Luteete and Mwanamugimu)*

		Percentage giving correct answer (shown in parentheses or italics)
DISEASE (reproducibility .84; scalability .52)		
When child small, should mother worry		78
Reasons why child stays small		58
Picture and description child, what disease		68
Too little staple or too little sauce		42
REARING (reproducibility .81; scalability .49)		
When introduce additional foods	(*4* or 6 months)	33
When wean	(14 or *18* months)	65
How many meals a day	(2 or *5* meals)	44
FOOD (reproducibility .91; scalability .51)		
Body-Building food?:		
milk	(yes)	86
matooke	(no)	66
'English' potatoes	(no)	13
paw-paw	(no)	9
SNACKS (reproducibility .94; scalability .65)		
Tea with milk or fruit juice		89
Orange or *egg*		70
Groundnuts or sweet banana		12

the age of 12 months, and to give a child at least three or four meals a day. During pretesting it was found that the women apparently picked up this information very quickly and that, once they had attended a few times, nearly all of them gave the correct answers. The questions were made slightly more difficult by having the respondents choose from two, both incorrect, answers – this is known as the error-choice technique (Hammond, 1948). The assumption is that one of these two answers indicates a greater insight than the other (Table 30). For example, with the question about the number of meals clearly one of the two alternatives (five meals) is the answer most closely reflecting the teaching. The percentages of 'best' answers are given in Table 30, with the coefficients resulting from Guttman scaling. In general, the women did not like this procedure, often replying that neither of the answers was correct.

Food knowledge

A third area of the teaching concerns foods. Widely used is the concept of body-building foods, to indicate foods with a relatively high protein content that are conducive to growth. The common staples, such as matooke and sweet potato, for example, are not considered to be body-building foods. This scale consists of the four answers to the questions whether the following were body-building foods: matooke (no), milk (yes), 'English' potatoes (no), and paw-paw (no). Results are again presented in Table 30. Surprisingly, of the mothers attending the clinic for the first time, the majority already know that matooke is not a body-building food. On the other hand, they widely regard 'English' potatoes and paw-paw as such.

Snacks knowledge

The teaching at the clinics concentrates predominantly on the foods that compose the main meals, but small children often eat and drink other things in between. This knowledge scale attempted to measure how far snacks or drinks relatively rich in protein (tea with milk, an egg, groundnuts) were regarded as more valuable than low-protein snacks (fruit juice, an orange, sweet bananas). The question that was asked was: 'Which of these two is better for a 2-year-old child?' The meaning of this scale is somewhat ambiguous, in that the low-protein snacks, particularly fruit juice and orange, have other nutritional qualities.

Summarizing, it can be said that the four knowledge scales are fairly homogeneous according to the coefficients of reproducibility and scalability in Table 30, although there are relatively few items within each scale.

B.2 Attitude scales: paired comparison method

This scaling technique was originally developed by Thurstone, and the statistical assumptions and calculation procedures have been described by Edwards (1957) and Kendall (1970). Respondents are asked to compare two stimuli, and to select which of them is preferable, according to certain criteria. For example, if the stimuli are foods, the respondent may be asked to select which of two foods is 'better' or has a higher food value, and so forth. Several stimuli are employed, all possible pairings of them are presented and from this an overall preference ranking may be established.

To gain insight into existing food preferences in Uganda, several pilot studies were carried out. People attending various health centres and dispensaries in Buganda were interviewed using different lists of foods. These interviews were conducted in Luganda with the help of a female interpreter. Subjects were asked to choose 'Which of these two foods would you prefer to feed to your two-year-old child?' No further criterion by which to make the choice was suggested. The interviews in general posed few difficulties: people chose readily, even those without small children.

Another aim of these pilot studies was to estimate the optimum length of the interview. The length of a paired comparison schedule varies with the number of stimuli that are included. For example, four stimuli require six comparisons; with five stimuli ten comparisons have to be made, while eight stimuli give 28 comparisons. We soon found that for use in verbal presentation seven or eight foods was the workable maximum.

Table 31. *Average number of choices for each of six staple foods (N=47)*

Matooke	4.23	Maize	1.78
Rice	3.02	Cassava	1.58
Sweet potato	2.97	Millet	1.29

Table 31 gives six staple food preferences obtained in a pilot study with a group of 47 people. Since each staple was compared with every other, the maximum number of times that one food could be chosen was five, the minimum 0. The figures in the table present the average number of times a meal was chosen.[26] There is clearly an overwhelming preference for plantain, but surprisingly rice takes second position, closely followed by sweet potato. Rice is particularly popular among people living in urban and peri-urban areas, something which has also been observed in other parts of Africa. Among the least preferred staple foods are the most nutritious, maize and millet, while cassava is rather unpopular in this part of Uganda.

Table 32 presents similar results, this time for six relishes. Again the maximum possible number of times one could be chosen is five, the minimum 0. The pattern of choices is less polarized than for the staple foods, but it is clear that the animal foods are generally preferred, with fish and chicken foremost and meat next (meat is usually served very tough, and is not very suitable for small children).

Further pilot tests with other sauces also showed that high-protein sauces were generally far preferred over sauces of low protein value, such as cabbage, green leaves, 'bean soup' or 'meat soup'[13]. This preference for high-protein, over low-protein, sauces posed a problem. Initially we had intended to select some high- and some low-protein sauces, and to find out whether with education preferences shifted towards the high-protein sauces. But since these were already so highly regarded, it would be difficult to demonstrate any further changes in that direction. Another possibility was to compare staples with sauces hoping that the teaching would show a shift in preference towards the sauces. Staple and sauce are, however, considered very distinct parts of the meal, and cannot be compared. When a number of people were asked to make such a comparison they either refused

Table 32. *Average number of choices for each of six sauces (N=90)*

Fish	3.23	Beans	2.59
Chicken	3.08	Groundnuts	1.84
Meat	2.68	Green vegetables	1.57

or said that it was ridiculous. Therefore complete meals had to be used as stimuli, that is, combinations of staple and sauce which differed in protein content. A highly regarded staple, matooke, was combined with three low-protein sauces, while a less popular staple, sweet potato, was combined with three high-protein sauces, six meals in all. The rationale for this was that the traditional choice would consider primarily the staple, hence would centre on the popular matooke meals, while recognition of the importance of protein sauces would encourage the respondent to choose the high-protein meals, despite the less favoured staple.

Six meals gave a total of 15 comparisons that had to be made. Two comparisons were included twice in the interview schedule to check on the reliability of choices. For the 97 mothers who were making their first visit to the clinics, 80 per cent gave an identical response on the repeat presentation. This is not perfect, but consistent enought to warrant further use. Table 33 presents the average number of choices for each meal for this group. Choices were evenly distributed between high- and low-protein meals, which suggests that the women were already taking both the staple food and the sauce into consideration. If they had based their choices only on the staple food, choices for the matooke meals should have predominated. One type of inaccuracy in the replies consists of 'circular triads' - apparent logical inconsistencies in the choices of an individual, which, in this case, were statistically removed.[27]

The index which will be called high-protein meals is based on the nine occasions when the three high-protein meals were compared with the three low-protein meals and represents the number of times the high-protein meals were preferred. A reliability coefficient[28] of .84 was computed for this measure in the group of first attenders. It was expected that with education the number of choices for high-protein meals would increase.

Table 33. *Average number of choices for each of six meals (N=97)*

Matooke with bean soup	3.3	Sweet potato with fish	3.6
Matooke with meat soup	1.4	Sweet potato with beans	2.8
Matooke with cabbage	2.8	Sweet potato with meat	1.1

B.3 Attitude scales: semantic differential

This rating method was developed by Osgood and his associates, and is described in *The Measurement of Meaning* (Osgood *et* al., 1957). Virtually any concept can be rated by this method, which uses contrasting adjectives such as 'good-bad', 'hard-soft', or 'fast-slow'. The respondent is asked to consider a certain concept (e.g. a food) and to indicate which of the two words best describes it, and also to what extent this word applies. For example, when he regards the concept as 'good' (vs 'bad'), a respondent indicates whether he considers it 'slightly' good, 'quite' good or even 'very' good as below:

Good			Neutral			Bad
very	quite	slightly		slightly	quite	very

By rating the concept against several such wordpairs, the respondent provides a profile of complementary ratings. These may, for example, demonstrate differences between concepts or individuals and may also illustrate changes over time.

Adjectives are selected according to their meanings and their relevance in describing a particular concept or group of concepts. An instrument of this type is known as a semantic differential, and has been used in different cultures. Osgood *et al.* (1957) reported that, independently of the concept being judged, people tend to make judgements on the basis of three different aspects or dimensions. These 'dimensions' were identified as *evaluation,* exemplified by wordpairs such as 'good-bad' or 'happy-sad'; *potency* which features wordpairs such as 'strong-weak' and 'hard-soft'; and *activity,* consisting of wordpairs such as 'active-passive' and 'fast-slow'. Individual scales may be aggregated within these three dimensions, making the results more concise.

Luganda version

The first step in developing a Luganda version was the selection of wordpairs. A list of adjectives was taken from Osgood *et al.* (1957, p. 53), and three interpreters, working independently, translated these into Luganda. Subsequently the Luganda opposites were written next to these words. The resulting wordpairs were translated back into English by one of the other translators. These translations were compared with the original adjective and its English opposite. (This opposite itself had also been included elsewhere in the list.) After reviewing the consistency of translation and re-translation, 23 pairs of Luganda adjectives were selected for further use covering the three dimensions previously mentioned (Table 34). As a result of this procedure both the Luganda and English meanings of the adjectives were well established. The next step was to determine on what dimensions they might best be grouped.

A group of 200 Baganda boys and girls in the senior forms of three secondary schools judged the similarity between the different words, according to a method proposed by Osgood *et al.* (1957, p. 39). Questionnaires were prepared in which two wordpairs had been printed on each line.

GOOD-bad happy-sad

The students indicated which word of the second pair (here, happy or sad) was most similar in meaning to the first word printed in capital letters. (The 23 wordpairs make 253 combinations, but each student was presented with about half of these, according to a random rotation system.) The idea behind this procedure is that if the two wordpairs are related and somewhat similar in meaning, one of the two words in the second pair will consistently be chosen. The degree to which this is the case reflects the degree to which the wordpairs are related. If they are totally unrelated, choices will be made randomly, and each word of the second pair will receive approximately 50 per cent of the choices.

In first instance, analysis had to be limited to visual inspection of the preference matrix. This suggested that there were not three, but two, basic dimensions - the first being evaluative, and the second a mixture of activity and potency. We therefore concentrated on these two dimensions in the further development of this scale. Later computer analysis produced four dimensions of which the first two are the most meaningful (Table 34). These include an evaluative dimension (but which also contains some activity scales), while the second dimension indicates mainly strength and difficulty. By and large, this confirms the decision to concentrate on only two dimensions.[29]

Table 34. *Kruskal multidimensional scaling, 23 wordpairs, 4 dimensions, stress 25 per cent*

	1	2	3	4
sweet - sour	.67	-.74	-	-
happy - sad	1.08	-	-	-
good - bad	.89	-	-	-
wise - foolish	1.10	-	-	-
right - wrong	.80	-	-	-
tasty - not tasty	.89	-.52	-	-
high - low	.62	.60	-.52	-
strong - weak	.53	.52	-	-
intentional - unintentional	.49	.30	.40	-.36
warm - cold	.85	.48	-.30	-.48
alive - dead	.87	-	.33	-
difficult - easy	-.48	.92	-	-
fast - slow	.86	-	-	.53
active - passive	.80	-	-	-
wide - narrow	.52	-	.57	.61
hard - soft	-.35	.95	-	-
long - short	.69	.69	-	.37
masculine - feminine	.30	.84	-	-
brave - cowardly	.74	.72	.39	-
heavy - light	-	.54	1.01	-
central - peripheral	.56	-	-	-.71
dry - wet	-	-.59	.81	-
usual - unusual	.48	-.60	-	-

Trial versions

Because some of the wordpairs were unsuitable for describing foods, they had to be omitted or replaced. Next, two contrasting groups of people were given the wordpairs on paper and asked to judge various foods. The first group consisted of 26 villagers while the second comprised 13 nurses at a baby home in Kampala-groups that might be expected to differ in attitudes towards foods. Results are presented in Figure 6. Allowing for the small number of respondents in the second group, there are consistent differences between the two groups, particularly on the activity and potency wordpairs (busy-idle, quick-slow, active-passive, strong-weak, heavy-light, and hard-soft). The nurses rate the staple food, matooke, consistently lower than do the rural respondents on these scales. The nurses also draw a greater contrast between the staple food and a legume than the villagers.

Final scale

Ten wordpairs were finally selected for further use (see Table 35). It was decided to use them in conjunction with two concepts, 'matooke', the local staple food, and 'enva', the Luganda word for 'sauce'. The expectation was that the rating of sauce (enva) would increase with education, while that of matooke should fall.

In studies at four teacher training colleges (see also Chapter 7) the scales were given to first- and fourth-year students, using seven-point scales and a paper and pencil application. Although the majority of the students were Baganda, Swahili and English translations of the wordpairs were also presented. The ratings for 'sauce' were uniformly very high and showed little variation but matooke was rated less positively, and these ratings also showed greater variation. Table 35 presents the results of a factor analysis of the matooke ratings. This analysis broadly confirms the previous results, and points to two basic factors. The first dimension includes six wordpairs, and is clearly 'evaluative'. The second consists of four wordpairs and includes activity and strength. The pair 'poor-rich' loads equally on both dimensions but given the other results it was decided to retain it in the evaluative dimension. To conclude, it can be said that in relation to food, the respondents apparently distinguished between an 'evaluative' and a 'dynamic' component, with the latter including aspects of 'potency' and 'activity'. In further analyses, scores obtained with the ten wordpairs were grouped into two indicators, the evaluative score obtained with the first six wordpairs and the dynamic score from adding together the scores on the last four wordpairs (Table 35).

When used with the mothers attending the clinics, the wordpairs were presented verbally, employing five-point ratings as described in the text.[30] Composite scores were computed for 97 mothers making their first visit to either Mwanamugimu or Luteete clinic (Figure 7). These frequency distributions show that

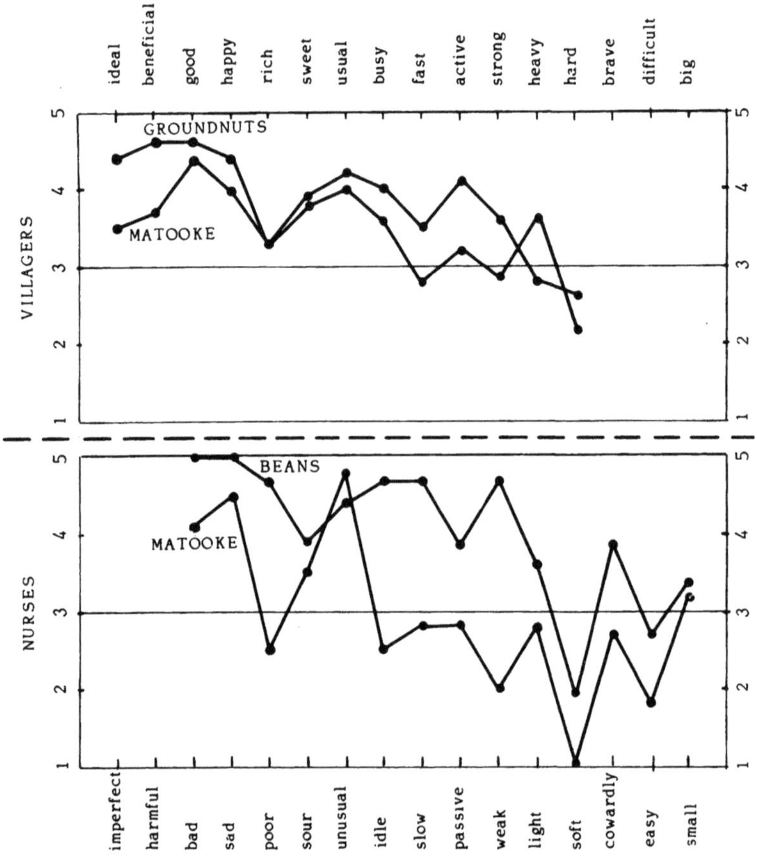

Figure 6. *Semantic differential: ratings of groups of villagers (N=26) and nurses (N=13)*

Table 35. *Semantic differential, judgements of concept 'Matooke': Varimax rotation of first two principal components (N=407)*

Luganda:	Loadings on dimension 1 'Evaluative'	Loadings on dimension 2 'Dynamic'	English equivalent
kisanyufu-kinakuwavu	.45	-.05	happy - sad
kyavu-kigagga	-.46	.46	poor - rich
kinene-kitono	.50	-.16	big - small
sikyamugaso-kyamugaso	-.73	.19	unimportant - important
yentufu-siyentufu	.70	-.21	ideal - imperfect
kibi-kirungi	-.78	.14	bad - good
kyamanyi-kinafu	.16	-.78	strong - weak
mpola-mangu	-.10	.50	slow - fast
kititizi-kizira	-.07	.74	cowardly - brave
mukozi-simukozi	.41	-.61	active - passive

the ratings of sauce were overwhelmingly positive, to such an extent that 67 per cent and 51 per cent of the respondents obtained the maximum score. The ratings for matooke, however, were less extreme, and here only 28 per cent and 15 per cent of the respondents achieved the maximum score.[31] The range of scores for matooke was also considerably larger than for sauce. Since there was hardly room for increases in the sauce ratings, they were excluded from further analysis; only the evaluative and the dynamic ratings of matooke were retained.

B.4 Validation

The previous sections of this appendix describe the development of four knowledge scales, one preference scale, (the high-protein meals), and two ratings resulting from the semantic differential. The selection of the items that were included in these instruments was done largely on the basis of considerations of internal consistency. However, since all seven scales are concerned with nutrition, they may be expected to correlate, to some extent, with

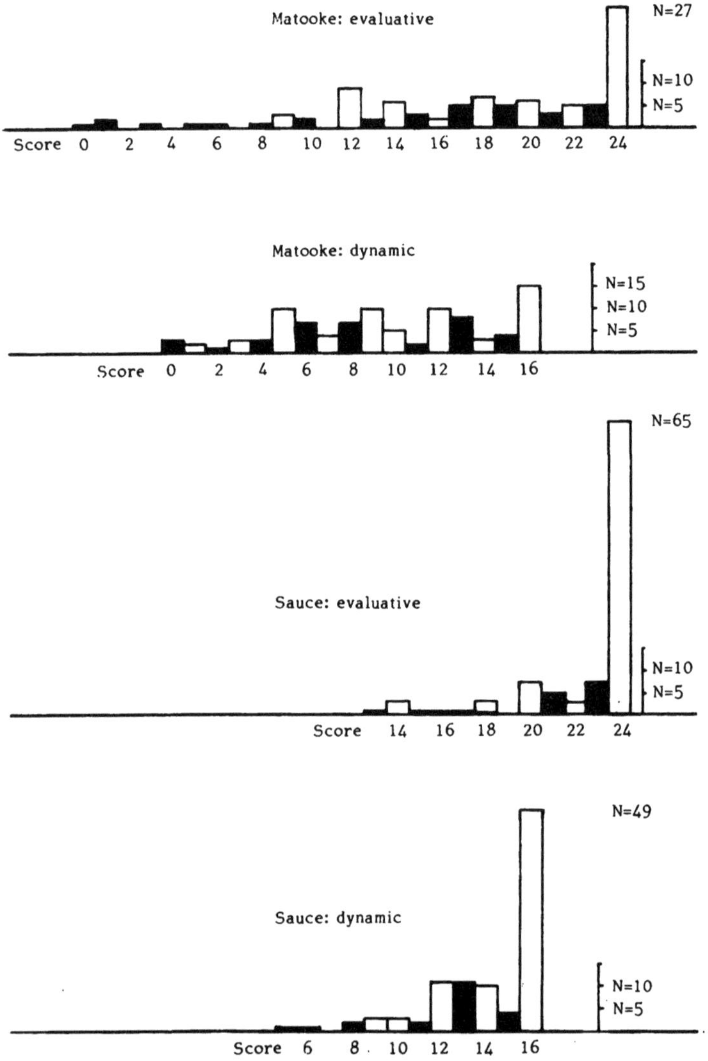

Figure 7. *Semantic differential: frequency distributions of four composite scores (first attenders, N=97)*

Table 36. *Spearman rank correlations between knowledge and attitude scales (first attenders, N=97)*

	1	2	3	4	5	6
1. Disease						
2. Child rearing	.12					
3. Food	.16*	.14				
4. Snacks	.05	-.03	.11			
5. High-protein meals	.24**	.10	.10	-.12		
6. Matooke: Evaluative	-.15	-.05	-.29**	.14	-.28**	
7. Matooke: Dynamic	-.20*	-.05	-.34**	.14	-.19	.74**

* $p<.05$
** $p<.01$

each other. The presence or absence of intercorrelations can be used as a criterion of validity. It was decided that for an indicator to be included in further analysis it should correlate significantly with at least one other indicator. If not, it was to be excluded. Table 36 presents these correlations computed for the 97 mothers who were interviewed when first attending the three clinics.

The two indicators that fall short of the criterion are the knowledge scales that centre around child rearing practices and preferences for snacks. It was mentioned that the rationale behind these two scales was somewhat farfetched, and from this matrix it appears to be unclear what they measure. The other five indicators show at least one statistically significant correlation while all of the correlations between them are in the expected directions. The knowledge scales concerned with disease and with foods and the number of high-protein meals chosen correlate positively among themselves. They correlate negatively with the ratings of matooke, which means that those who do rate matooke highly score lower on the other scales. The two ratings, evaluative and dynamic, correlate highly with each other, which may indicate that these first attenders draw little distinction between these two aspects.

Notes

1. During 1974 an administrative reorganization of regions and districts took place, but since most of the literature uses the previous boundaries, these will be retained here.
2. The information in this section was taken from *Atlas of Uganda* (1967) and Langlands (1974).
3. The percentages for the five districts were: Busoga 1.3, Bukedi 1.2, Bugisu 0.9, Kigezi 0.9, and Ankole 0.5 per cent. The percentages that are actually reported by Dean and Burgess (1962) are all ten times higher but it appears that an error was made in connection with the decimal point. The percentages presented here were calculated from the raw figures, given by Burgess (1962, a,b,c,d,e), expressing as a percentage the total number of observed cases by the number of children older than 8 months and younger than 5 years of age.
4. The percentages for the nine districts were as follows: Busoga 7.0, Bukedi 14.5, Bugisu 5.6, Kigezi 6.4, Mengo 11.2, Masaka 5.4, Mubende 17.6, Bunyoro 8.7, and Toro 4.7 per cent.
5. The work in the rural health centres seemed to have little attraction for these young women. Of about 40 assistant health visitors who qualified from the two courses each year it seems that less than half joined the staff of health centres in rural areas. Others took up places in government hospitals, mission hospitals, or in local administration. Among those assistant health visitors who did start working in a rural area there tended to be a rapid turnover. They married or moved to urban areas, where they often joined the staff of a hospital. Although hospitals employ assistant health visitors to give health education in all wards, it seems that most of them sooner or later took up regular nursing duties.
6. Detailed information is contained in reports by Cook (1967) and Moffat (1969).
7. For convenience all female attendants with children are called 'mothers', unless indicated otherwise.

8. The title of such centres varies from country to country: they may also be known as Mothercraft Centres or Nutrition Rehabilitation Units, and they have many similarities with the broader-scope Applied Nutrition Programmes (F.A.O./W.H.O., 1966).
9. The name of the centre is derived from a local, Ganda proverb *Mwanamugimu ava ku ngozi,* meaning 'the beautiful flower comes from good roots'. This suggests, by analogy, that the healthy child is one who comes from a good and caring home.
10. It is interesting to note that the previously reported finding that some 25 per cent of the outpatients at Mwanamugimu did not make adequate progress has also been reported from other countries. Bengoa in his review concluded that 'In most nutritional rehabilitation centres about 20-25% of the children do not improve in spite of a satisfactory diet given over a period of several months' (Bengoa, 1976, p. 327). See also Roemer (1972) and Beghin and Viteri (1973) for general discussions.
11. The terms used here follow the suggestions of Campbell and Stanley (1966); the reader is reminded that other authors occasionally use similar terms but for different designs.
12. If records of reattendances are kept at the clinic an alternative procedure exists for the selection of a control group. A random group of first attenders is selected and studied. Later, when a suitable period of time has passed, only those cases are retained for analysis that have reattended as required, while the cases that have failed to return are rejected.
13. 'Bean soup' and 'meat soup' consist of the water in which beans or meat have been cooked, and contain very little actual beans or meat. They are often used for children but are also eaten by adults, even being offered cheaply in local restaurants.
14. Many children in the group of first attenders at Luteete were younger than 6 months. Before that age most African children are still on the breast and of reasonable nutritional status, while those who decline usually do so after that age. Had these children been included in the control group at Luteete, a distorted picture would have resulted showing a relative decline in nutritional status with attendance at Luteete. Instead the average nutritional status was computed only for those children that were 6 months of age or older when they first attended. This is the reason for the small size of the Luteete control group in this instance.
15. Of course, it can also be argued that one aim of the teaching should be that people learn to make more refined judgements. The results indicate that this does not happen.
16. Contrary to the selection procedure of the first study, no upper limit was imposed on the number of visits, with the aim of increasing the number of available subjects.
17. For that reason inconsistencies in the answers were, in this case, not removed, in contrast to the previous study (see Note 27).
18. For those readers who are familiar with the problems of quantifying paired comparison data, it must be emphasized that the protein index and the

staple index are independent measures although they are both computed from the same paired-comparison schedule.

19. It seems that, among the Baganda, the staff selects for admission as inpatients those women who are least conscious of the protein content of different meals. A similar finding was noted in Chapter 5, page 67.
20. A further breakdown of scores showed that the results for boys and girls were very much the same, and that there certainly is no difference in trends between the colleges for girls and the colleges for boys.
21. The role of weaning in the causation of malnutrition is not discussed here, because, by its nature, it no longer plays a role during recovery. A brief discussion can be found in Hoorweg (1976, pp. 13-14).
22. 17 shillings (Uganda) = £ 1 Sterling at 1972 exchange rates.
23. Interview schedule: Study 5.

Diet

Var 1 Is the food for the child prepared and served according to the recommended methods?

1 = no
2 = sometimes) cooked separately, but not mashed
3 = always
4 = sometimes) cooked separately and mashed.
5 = always

Var 2 Child's appetite.

1 = refuses food regularly
2 = refuses food when ill
3 = never refuses food

Resources

Var 3 Land available to the household.

1 = none
2 = one plot held permanently or temporary tenure of one plot or more
3 = more than one plot held permanently

Var 4 Cash incomes; number of different sources.
(range 0-3)

Food resources

Var 5 Foods grown; number of different crops grown, excluding staple foods.
(range 0-3)

Var 6 Foods bought; expenditure.

1 = none
2 = 29 shillings or less per week
3 = 30 shillings or more per week

Var 7 Availability of milk.
1 = none
2 = only when provided by Mwanamugimu clinic
3 = bought occasionally
4 = have their own cows

Mother's knowledge and attitudes
Var 8 Education; form reached.
1 = none and primary 1
2 = primary 2
etc. (straight count)

Var 9 Number of visits to the clinic
(straight count)

Var 10 Attitude score.
(range 0-9)

Household situation
Var 11 Family situation.
1 = mother not married and living on her own
2 = husband works elsewhere, and returns home irregularly
3 = married, husband absent
4 = unmarried, living with family
5 = married, living with husband

Var 12 Number of people in the household. (straight count up to 11, anything above coded 12)

Support from others
Var 13 Help with household activities.
0 = none
1 = part-time farm labourer
2 = full-time farm labourer
3 = family member
4 = farm labourer + family member

Var 14 Attitude of husband towards the teaching of Mwanamugimu
0 = disagrees
1 = indifferent
2 = agrees
3 = not discussed
4 = encourages to implement
5 = actively helps to implement

Var 15 Attitude of relatives towards the teaching of Mwanamugimu
(as var 14)

Tribe

Var 16 Mother; comes originally from:
1 = Sudan
2 = North Uganda
3 = Kenya, Tanzania
4 = Rwanda, Burundi, or belongs to a tribe which has plantain as the predominant staple food
5 = Basoga, Banyoro, Wakiga, Banyankole
6 = Baganda

24. Since most of the variables have nonparametric distributions, single correlations were computed according to the Spearman formula. Because Spearman correlations, in general, give fair estimates of underlying Pearson correlations, multiple correlations were calculated from these correlations with the help of the formula by Pearson (Guilford, 1965).
25. Presently a research team of the Afrika-Studiecentrum is stationed in Kenya to study the relationship between nutrition intervention and environment. Information about this project can be obtained from Hoorweg through the Afrika-Studiecentrum.
26. It has been customary to convert these scores into scale values with the help of z-distributions (Edwards, 1957), but it has been shown that this, in the majority of cases, is an unnecessary procedure (Scott, 1968).
27. A circular triad occurs when a subject prefers A over B; and B over C; but instead of choosing A over C, as could be expected, she chooses C. Circular triads can be regarded as mere errors of judgement, but may as well reflect genuine changes in the criteria used from comparison to comparison. In this case it was decided to treat circular triads as errors because neither their total number - statistically tested following Kendall (1970) - nor their distribution over subjects and items indicated a systematic pattern.

    For further analysis, the circular triads were removed from the data by use of a weighting procedure described by Kendall (1955), a procedure which amounts to a repeated application of the Sonnenborg-Berner scoring system, well known to chess players. The resulting order of preferences is the best possible estimation of the true order underlying the actual choices.
28. KR20, with correction for variations in item difficulty (Horst, 1953).
29. There has been a long-standing debate about the existence of separate evaluation, potency, and activity dimensions. Although the wordpairs that make up the evaluative factor are the same in many different cultures, it has also been found that the wordpairs which make up the potency and activity factors vary the more the languages are removed from the Western European group of languages, findings which accord with our own (see Osgood, May, and Miron, 1975).
30. Previous attempts to apply seven-point scales, with the help of visual aids, had failed.
31. These results do not confirm one of the premises implicit in the teaching, that people are generally unaware of the value of the sauces.

References

Ainsworth, M. D. (1967). *Infancy in Uganda.* Baltimore: Johns Hopkins Press.

Albino, R. C., & Thompson, V. J. (1956). The effects of sudden weaning on Zulu children. *British Journal of Medical Psychology,* 29, 177-210.

Ashworth, A. (1969). Growth rates in children recovering from protein-energy malnutrition. *British Journal of Nutrition,* 23, 835-45.

Ashworth, A., Bell, R., James, W. P. T., & Waterlow, J. C. (1968). Calorie requirements of children recovering from protein-calorie malnutrition. *Lancet,* (2), 600-603.

Atlas of Uganda (2nd ed.) (1967). Uganda Government, Department of Land and Surveys.

Bain, K. (1973). Introduction. In D. B. Jelliffe & E. B. Jelliffe (Eds.), *Nutrition programmes for preschool children,* pp. 5-6. Zagreb: Institute of Public Health.

Beaudry-Darismé, M., & Latham, M. C. (1973). Nutritional rehabilitation centres: An evaluation of their performance. *Journal of Tropical Pediatrics and Environmental Child Health,* 19, 299-332.

Beghin, I. D. (1970). Nutrition rehabilitation centers in Latin America: A critical assessment. *American Journal of Clinical Nutrition,* 23, 1412-17.

Beghin, I. D. (1972). Improvement of the nutritional status of infants and children - consideration of Northeast Brazil program. In *Proceedings of the Western Hemisphere Nutrition Congress III,* pp. 93-8. New York: Futura.

Beghin, I. D., & Viteri, F. E. (1973). Nutritional rehabilitation centers: An evaluation of their performance. *Journal of Tropical Pediatrics and Environmental Child Health,* 19, 404-16.

Bengoa, J. M. (1964). Nutrition rehabilitation programmes. *Journal of Tropical Pediatrics,* 10, 63-4.

Bengoa, J. M. (1967). Nutrition rehabilitation centres. *Journal of Tropical Pediatrics,* 13, 169-76.

Bengoa, J. M. (1973). Significance of malnutrition and priorities for its prevention. In A. Berg, N. S. Scrimshaw, & D. L. Call (Eds.), *Nutrition, national development, and planning,* pp. 103-28. Cambridge, Mass.: M.I.T. Press.

Bengoa, J. M. (1976). Nutritional rehabilitation. In G. H. Beaton & J. M. Bengoa (Eds.), *Nutrition in preventive medicine,* pp. 321-34. Geneva: World Health Organization, monograph 62.

Bengoa, J. M., & Beaton, G. H. (1976). Some concepts and practical considerations in planning and evaluation. In G. H. Beaton & J. M. Bengoa (Eds.), *Nutrition in preventive medicine,* pp. 213-22. Geneva: World Health Organization, monograph 62.

Bennett, F. J., Lutwama, J. S. W., & Namboze, J. (1963). What Baganda men want to know . . . *International Journal of Health Education,* 6, 192-7.

Bennett, F. J., & Stanfield, J. P. (1971). The clinical conditions and aetiology of malnutrition in Uganda. *Journal of Tropical Pediatrics and Environmental Child Health,* 17, monograph 13, 5-10.

Berg, A. (1973). *The nutrition factor.* Washington: Brookings Institution.

Berggren, W. L. (1971). Evaluation of the effectiveness of education and rehabilitation centers. In *Proceedings of the Western Hemisphere Nutrition Congress III,* pp. 34-7. New York: Futura.

Blankhart, D. M. (1971). Outline for a survey of the feeding and the nutritional status of children under three years of age and their mothers. *Journal of Tropical Pediatrics and Environmental Child Health,* 17, 175-86.

Bosley, B. (1976). Nutrition education. In G. H. Beaton & J. M. Bengoa (Eds.), *Nutrition in preventive medicine,* pp. 277-96. Geneva: World Health Organization, monograph 62.

Brown, R. E., & Opio, E. A. (1966). Associated factors in kwashiorkor in Uganda. *Tropical and Geographical Medicine,* 18, 119-24.

Burgess, H. J. L. (1962a). Protein-calorie malnutrition in Uganda: Busoga district. *East African Medical Journal,* 39, 362-74.

Burgess, H. J. L. (1962b). Protein-calorie malnutrition in Uganda: Bukedi district. *East African Medical Journal,* 39, 375-85.

Burgess, H. J. L. (1962c). Protein-calorie malnutrition in Uganda: Bugisu district. *East African Medical Journal,* 39, 386-90.

Burgess, H. J. L. (1962d). Protein-calorie malnutrition in Uganda: Ankole district. *East African Medical Journal,* 39, 391-400.

Burgess, H. J. L. (1962e). Protein-calorie malnutrition in Uganda: Kigezi district. *East African Medical Journal,* 39, 401-10.

Burgess, H. J. L., & Burgess, A. P. (1972). Nutritional content and value of local foodstuffs: A critical appraisal. In V. F. Amann, D. G. R. Belshaw & J. P. Stanfield (Eds.), *Nutrition and food in an African economy, volume 1,* pp. 45-58. Kampala: Makerere University, Department of Rural Economy.

Campbell, D. T., & Stanley, J. C. (1966). *Experimental and quasi-experimental designs for research.* Chicago: Rand McNally.

Church, M. A., & Stanfield, J. P. (1971). The weight chart: An invaluable aid in nutrition rehabilitation. *Journal of Tropical Pediatrics and Environmental Child Health,* 17, monograph 13, 61-6.

Cleave, J. H. (1972). Food requirements and availability in Uganda: A national food balance sheet. In V. F. Amann, D. G. R. Belshaw & J. P. Stanfield (Eds.), *Nutrition and food in an African economy, volume 1,* pp. 109-25. Kampala:

Makerere University, Department of Rural Economy.
Cook, R. (1967). *The Ankole pre-school protection programme.* Mimeographed report.
Cook, R. (1971). Is hospital the place for the treatment of malnourished children? *Journal of Tropical Pediatrics and Environmental Child Health,* 17, 15-25.
Dean, R. F. A., & Burgess, H. J. L. (1962). Protein-calorie malnutrition in Uganda: Conclusions of the survey and recommendations. *East African Medical Journal,* 39, 411-16.
De Mayer, E. M. (1976). Protein-energy malnutrition. In G. H. Beaton & J. M. Bengoa (Eds.), *Nutrition in preventive medicine,* pp. 23-54. Geneva: World Health Organization, monograph 62.
Edwards, A. L. (1957). *Techniques of attitude scale construction.* New York: Appleton-Century-Crofts.
Eisler, M., Ravines, L. C., & Ramirez, J. L. (1969). The nutrition rehabilitation center. *Journal of the American Dietetic Association,* 55, 246-51.
Elinson, J. (1967). Effectiveness of social action programs in health and welfare. In A. B. Bergman (Ed.), *Assessing the effectiveness of child health services,* pp. 77-81. Columbus: Ross Laboratories. Reprinted in C. H. Weiss (Ed.), *Evaluating action programs: Readings in social action and education,* pp. 294-9. Boston: Allyn and Bacon, 1972.
F.A.O./W.H.O. (1966). *Report of the joint F.A.O./W.H.O. technical meeting on methods of planning and evaluation in applied nutrition programmes.* Rome: Food and Agricultural Organization, nutrition meetings report no. 39.
F.A.O./W.H.O. (1976). *Food and nutrition strategies in national development.* Rome: Food and Agriculture Organization, nutrition meetings report no. 56.
Farmer, A. P. (1960). Malnutrition as an ecological problem. *East African Medical Journal,* 37, 399-404.
Frood, J. D. L., Whitehead, R. G., & Coward, W. A. (1971). Relationship between pattern of infection and development of hypoalbuminaemia and hypo-β-lipoproteinaemia in rural Ugandan children. *Lancet,* (2), 1047-9.
Garrow, J. S., & Pike, M. C. (1967). The short term prognosis of severe primary infantile malnutrition. *British Journal of Nutrition,* 21, 155-65.
Gongora, J., & McFie, J. (1959). Malnutrition, malaria and mortality: The use of a simple questionnaire in an epidemiological study. *Transactions of the Royal Society of Tropical Medicine and Hygiene,* 53, 238-47.
Gordon, J. E. (1976). Synergism of malnutrition and infectious disease. In G. H. Beaton & J. M. Bengoa (Eds.), *Nutrition in preventive medicine,* pp. 193-209. Geneva: World Health Organization, monograph 62.
Gordon, J. E., & Scrimshaw, N. S. (1973). Field evaluation of nutrition intervention programs. *World Review of Nutrition and Dietetics,* 17, 1-38.
Graham, G. G., Cordano, A., Blizzard, R. M., & Cheek, D. B. (1969). Infantile malnutrition: Changes in body composition during rehabilitation. *Pediatric Research,* 3, 579-89.
Green, L. W., & Figá-Talamanca, I. (1974). Suggested designs for evaluation of patient education programs. *Health Education Monographs,* 2, 54-70.
Guilford, J. P. (1965). *Fundamental statistics in psychology and education.* 4th edition. New York: McGraw-Hill.

Hammond, K. R. (1948). Measuring attitudes by error-choice: An indirect method. *Journal of Abnormal and Social Psychology,* 43, 38-48.
Harrison, D. W. (1972). Launching a non-imported nutritional supplement: The African Basic Food pilot scheme. In V. F. Amann, D. G. R. Belshaw, & J. P. Stanfield (Eds.), *Nutrition and food in an African economy, volume 1,* pp. 325-34. Kampala: Makerere University, Department of Rural Economy.
Hay, R. W., Whitehead, R. G., & Spicer, C. C. (1975). Serum-albumin as a prognostic indicator in oedematous malnutrition. *Lancet,* (2), 427-9.
Hoorweg, J. (1976). *Protein-energy malnutrition and intellectual abilities.* The Hague-Paris: Mouton Publishers.
Hoorweg, J., & Stanfield, J. P. (1976). The effects of protein-energy malnutrition in early childhood on intellectual and motor abilities in later childhood and adolescence. *Developmental Medicine and Child Neurology,* 18, 330-50.
Horst, P. (1953). Correcting the Kuder-Richardson reliability for dispersion of item difficulties. *Psychological Bulletin,* 50, 371-4.
Houston, T. R. (1972). The behavioral sciences impact-effectiveness model. In P. H. Rossi & W. Williams (Eds.), *Evaluating social programs: Theory, practice, and politics,* pp. 51-65. New York: Seminar Press.
Jelliffe, D. B. (1966). *The assessment of the nutritional status of the community.* Geneva: World Health Organization, monograph 53.
Jelliffe, D. B., & Dean, R. F. A. (1959). Protein-calorie malnutrition in early childhood. *Journal of Tropical Paediatrics and African Child Health,* 5, 96-106.
Jelliffe, D. B., Bennett, F. J., Stroud, C. E., Novotny, M. E., Karrach, H. A., Musoke, L. K., & Jelliffe, E. F. P. (1961). Field survey of the health of Bachiga children in the Kayinza district of Kigezi, Uganda. *American Journal of Tropical Medicine and Hygiene,* 10, 435-45.
Jelliffe, D. B., Bennett, F. J., White, R. H. R., Cullinan, T. R., & Jelliffe, E. F. P. (1962). The children of the Lugbara: A study in the techniques of paediatric field survey in tropical Africa. *Tropical and Geographical Medicine,* 14, 33-50.
Jelliffe, D. B., Bennett, F. J., Stroud, C. E., Welbourn, H. F., Williams, M. C., & Jelliffe, E. F. P. (1963). The health of Acholi children. *Tropical and Geographical Medicine,* 15, 411-21.
Jelliffe, D. B., Bennett, F. J., Jelliffe, E. F. P., & White, R. H. R. (1964). Ecology of childhood disease in the Karamojong of Uganda. *Archives of Environmental Health,* 9, 25-36.
Jelliffe, D. B., & Stanfield, J. P. (1966). Protein deficiencies and calorie deficiencies. *Lancet,* (2) 907-8.
Kendall, M. G. (1955). Further contributions to the theory of paired comparisons. *Biometrics,* 11, 43-62.
Kendall, M. G. (1970). *Rank correlation methods,* 4th edition. London: Griffin.
King, K. W. (1970). Mothercraft centers. *Nutrition Reviews,* 28, 307-9.
King, M. H., King, F. M. A., Morley, D. C., Burgess, H. J. L., & Burgess, A. P. (1972). *Nutrition for developing countries.* Nairobi: Oxford University Press.
Krieger, I., & Chen, Y. C. (1969). Calorie requirements for weight gain in infants with growth failure due to maternal deprivation, under-nutrition, and congenital heart disease. *Pediatrics,* 44, 647-54.

Langlands, B. W. (1974). *Atlas of population census 1969 in Uganda.* Occasional paper no. 48. Kampala: Makerere University, Department of Geography.
Latham, M. C. (1972). *Planning and evaluation of applied nutrition programmes.* Rome: Food and Agricultural Organization, nutritional studies no. 26.
Mandeville, E. (1974). *Failure and conformity in an African city.* Ph.D. thesis, Sussex University.
May, J. M., & McLellan, D. L. (1970). *The ecology of malnutrition in Eastern Africa and four countries of Western Africa.* New York: Hafner.
McDowell, I., & Clayden, D. (1974). Measuring the recovery rates of malnourished children from their weight-gains. Part 1: Review of existing methods. *Journal of Tropical Pediatrics and Environmental Child Health,* 25, 251-5.
McDowell, I., & Hoorweg, J. (1977). Environmental risk factors in outpatient recovery from malnutrition. *Journal of the Ecology of Food and Nutrition,* 6, 23-30.
McDowell, J. (1972). Patterns of protein availability and utilisation in Uganda. In V. F. Amann, D. G. R. Belshaw, & J. P. Stanfield (Eds.), *Nutrition and food in an African economy, volume I,* pp. 126-54. Kampala: Makerere University, Department of Rural Economy.
Moffat, M. (1969). *Mobile young child clinics in rural Uganda.* Mimeographed report.
Osgood, C. E. (1965). Cross-cultural comparability in attitude measurement via multilingual semantic differentials. In I. D. Steiner & M. Fishbein (Eds.), *Current studies in social psychology,* pp. 95-107. New York: Holt, Rinehart & Winston.
Osgood, C. E., May, W. H., & Miron, M. S. (1975). *Cross-cultural universals of affective meaning.* Urbana: University of Illinois Press.
Osgood, C. E., Suci, G. J., & Tannenbaum, P. H. (1957). *The measurement of meaning.* Urbana: University of Illinois Press.
Prader, A., Tanner, J. M., & von Harnack, G. A. (1963). Catch-up growth following illness or starvation. *Journal of Pediatrics,* 62, 646-59.
Rao, K. S. J. (1974). Evolution of kwashiorkor and marasmus. *Lancet,* (1), 709-11.
Robinson, D. C. (1971). The nutrition rehabilitation centre at Mulago Hospital, Kampala: Further development and evaluation, 1967-1969. *Journal of Tropical Pediatrics and Environmental Child Health,* 17, monograph 13, 35-42.
Roemer, M. I. (1972). *Evaluation of community health centres.* Geneva: World Health Organization, public health paper no. 48.
Rossi, P. H. (1972). Testing for success and failure in social action. In P. H. Rossi & W. Williams (Eds.), *Evaluating social programs: Theory, practice, and politics,* pp. 11-49. New York: Seminar Press.
Rutishauser, I. H. E. (1971). Statistics of malnutrition in early childhood. *Journal of Tropical Pediatrics and Environmental Child Health,* 17, monograph 13, 11-16.
Rutishauser, I. H. E., & Whitehead, R. G. (1969). Field evaluation of two biochemical tests which may reflect nutritional status in three areas of Uganda. *British Journal of Nutrition,* 23, 1-13.

Schneideman, I., Bennett, F. J., & Rutishauser, I. H. E. (1971). The nutrition rehabilitation unit at Mulago Hospital, Kampala: Development and evaluation, 1965-1967. *Journal of Tropical Pediatrics and Environmental Child Health,* 17, monograph 13, 25-34.

Scotney, N. (1976). *Health education.* Nairobi: African Medical and Research Foundation.

Scott, W. A. (1968). Attitude measurement. In G. Lindzey & E. Aronson (Eds.), *The handbook of social psychology; Volume 2: Research methods,* (2nd ed.), pp. 204-73. Reading, Mass: Addison-Wesley.

Sharman, A. (1972). Food consumption patterns in Eastern Uganda: A case study. In V. F. Amann, D. G. R. Belshaw, & J. P. Stanfield (Eds.), *Nutrition and food in an African economy, volume 1,* pp. 70-94. Kampala: Makerere University, Department of Rural Economy.

Southall, A. (1961). *Social change in modern Africa.* London: Oxford University Press.

Ssebaduka, L. C., & Goode, P. (1972). The Gayaza farm and diet scheme. In V. F. Amann, D. G. R. Belshaw, & J. P. Stanfield (Eds.), *Nutrition and food in an African economy, volume 1,* pp. 310-13. Kampala: Makerere University, Department of Rural Economy.

Stanfield, J. P. (1971). The Luteete family health centre: Nutrition rehabilitation as part of total rural development: An initial experience. *Journal of Tropical Pediatrics and Environmental Child Health,* 17, monograph 13, 67-82.

Suchman, E. A. (1967). *Evaluative research: Principles and practice in public service and social action programs.* New York: Russell Sage Foundation.

Uganda Government (1972). *Third five-year development plan, 1971/2-1975/6.*

Weiss, C. H. (1972). *Evaluation research: Methods of assessing program effectiveness.* Englewoods Cliffs, N. J.: Prentice-Hall.

Welbourn, H. F. (1955). The danger period during weaning. *Journal of Tropical Pediatrics,* (1), 34-46; (1), 98-111; (1), 161-73.

Welbourn, H. F. (1959). Backgrounds and follow-up of children with kwashiorkor. *Journal of Tropical Pediatrics,* 5, 84-95.

Welbourn, H. F. (1963). Custom and child health in Buganda: Methods of child rearing. *Tropical and Geographical Medicine,* 15, 124-33.

Wharton, B. (1971). The mortality of malnutrition in early childhood in Uganda. *Journal of Tropical Pediatrics and Environmental Child Health,* 17, monograph 13, 17-24.

W.H.O. (1974). Health education: A review of the W.H.O. programme. *W.H.O. Chronicle,* 28, 401-9.

Wober, M. (1974). Towards an understanding of the Kiganda concept of intelligence. In J. W. Berry and P. R. Dasen (Eds.), *Culture and cognition: Readings in cross-cultural psychology,* pp. 261-80. London: Methuen.

Young, F. A. (1972). The agricultural and nutrition project of the Uganda Company. In V. F. Amann, D. G. R. Belshaw, & J. P. Stanfield (Eds.), *Nutrition and food in an African economy, volume 1,* pp. 320-1. Kampala: Makerere University, Department of Rural Economy.

Already published
Jan Hoorweg

Protein-Energy Malnutrition and Intellectual Abilities

A study of teen-age Ugandan children

The question of whether protein-energy malnutrition during early childhood has a lasting influence on intellectual abilities carries grave social implications and has been the subject of a debate in medical and psychological circles during the last ten years. There is considerable difference of opinion among scientists, which to a large extent is a result of the weaknesses inherent in studies in this field, weaknesses of which the author first gives a critical analysis. Next, the results of a study among teen-age Ugandan children who had suffered severe malnutrition in early childhood are presented. Apart from intellectual abilities, motor development and daily behaviour of these children were also studied. On the basis of these findings, the author develops a theoretical framework which also accommodates the sometimes seemingly contradictory findings of the studies in other countries. It is shown that the long-term process of chronic malnutrition is a crucial factor affecting the child's intellectual development.

Communications 5, 1976, XVIII + 148 pages. Pb.
ISBN: 90-279-7752-6

Publication in collaboration with
AFRIKA-STUDIECENTRUM · LEIDEN

MOUTON PUBLISHERS · THE HAGUE · PARIS · NEW YORK

Bei Fragen zur Produktsicherheit wenden Sie sich bitte an:
If you have any questions regarding product safety,
please contact:

Walter de Gruyter GmbH
Genthiner Straße 13
10785 Berlin
productsafety@degruyterbrill.com